# REBEL FOR LIFE

*Rebel for Life: Breaking the Cycle of Weight Regain for Good*
Copyright © 2023 Cristy Nickel

This book is set in the typeface *Athelas* designed by Veronika Burian and Jose Scaglione.

Paperback ISBN: 978-1-955546-59-1

A Publication of *Tall Pine Books*
119 E Center Street, Suite B4A | Warsaw, Indiana 46580
*www.tallpinebooks.com*

| 1 23 23 20 16 02 |

Published in the United States of America

# REBEL FOR LIFE

## BREAKING THE CYCLE OF WEIGHT REGAIN FOR GOOD

### CRISTY "CODE RED" NICKEL

# CONTENTS

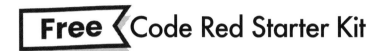 **Code Red Starter Kit**

*Download your free gift!*

Ready to jump-start your weight loss on the Code Red Lifestyle?
Grab your FREE Code Red Starter Kit now!

Your Starter Kit includes:

- Foods to Eat/Foods to Avoid List
- Weight/Water/Sleep Tracking Sheet
- Rules for Consistent Weight Loss

*Here's how to get your Code Red Starter Kit:*

✔ Head to www.CodeRedLifestyle.com/Print.
✔ Tell me where to email your Starter Kit.
✔ Check your email and download your three PDFs.
✔ Start taking your life back!

# THE CODE RED REBEL MANIFESTO

You are extraordinary! Do you know that?

The media, the food industry, the diet industry...

They all want you to believe there's something wrong with you. That you don't have any willpower.

That you have the wrong genetics. That you'll never be enough.

But you are strong.

And you're invited to STAND AND JOIN OUR REVOLUTION. We're taking back our lives, and we're doing it our own way. Thousands of men and women who say NO MORE!

WE'RE REBELLING against pills, powders, shakes, GMOs, low-fat, artificial ingredients, manufactured franken-foods.

WE'RE REBELLING against the people who say, "It's genetic. You'll always be fat."

WE'RE REBELLING against the diet industry, which is always trying to convince you there's something wrong with you and that this pill or that shake will fix it, if you'll just spend enough money.

WE'RE REBELLING against anyone or anything (especially yourself) that makes you hate your perfect, beautiful body!

WE'RE REBELLING against the external search for willpower. You already have all the power you'll ever need inside you!

And WE'RE JOINING TOGETHER to offer support when one Rebel stumbles or feels weak.

We are TAKING THE POWER BACK.

We are FINALLY TAKING CONTROL OF OUR OWN LIVES!

NO ONE gets to tell us what we should look like—not the TV, not magazines, not YouTube, not the insurance companies or the government.

NO ONE has the right to make us feel bad about our progress. Or tell us that we're doing it wrong.

Or assume that we're going to just "gain it all back."

No matter who you were before you joined the revolution, you are a new person now. You are whole and perfect and strong. You are a Code Red Rebel.

YOU CAN OVERCOME ANY CHALLENGE THAT STANDS IN YOUR WAY.

YOU CAN ACHIEVE YOUR GOALS.

WE BELIEVE IN YOU!

# DEAR READER

YOU'RE ABOUT TO read your last weight-loss book. If you choose to go on this journey with me, you WILL get your life back. People from all walks of life and all kinds of limiting circumstances have done it before you. But before we get started, I want to give you a sneak peek into what we're about to do together.

We don't have a weight loss problem in the modern world, we have a weight regain problem.

The Code Red Lifestyle has proven over and over again that anyone can lose weight without pills, powders, shakes or even exercise. My first book, *The Code Red Revolution*, went over how to do that in great detail. And tens of thousands of success stories prove how well it works.

We'll cover the lifestyle again briefly in this book, just to make sure you've got it. But what this book is REALLY designed to do is to help you understand how and why weight regain happens. This really is the last time you ever have to worry about your weight. If you choose, this can truly be the LAST time you go around this mountain.

There's nothing more frustrating to me than watching someone work so hard to lose 20, 50, or even 150 pounds, only to gain it back. It breaks my heart because I know what's going through their heads...

*What's wrong with me?*

*Why did I let this happen again?*

*I thought I had this thing licked!*

*I must be the dumbest person alive.*

*I'm such a loser.*

*I hate myself (still!)*

Hear me right now...

It's not your fault that you got heavy in the first place.

And there are absolutely ways to make sure you never get heavy again.

Your body is designed to survive. It's perfectly balanced to automatically behave in certain ways whenever certain conditions exist; conditions like fear, sadness, anger, boredom...and also conditions like joy, excitement, and celebration. It's funny how we can resort to eating to deal with both positive and negative emotions. From a survival standpoint, it makes total sense. By the end of this book, you will understand exactly what's happening and how you can consciously create a different outcome.

It doesn't matter how old you are.

It doesn't matter how much money you have.

It doesn't matter what you think your limitations are.

It doesn't matter if you've lost and regained weight dozens of times in the past...*this time will be different.*

You already have the power. All you need is to shine a light on what's happening on the INSIDE. If that sounds a little too woo-woo for you, let me assure you that this is all science. I'm a spiritual person, but I'm not going to ask God to magically keep me thin. Instead, I'm going to help you work WITH your body to keep you healthy and trim.

You can do this. I promise.

But once you learn this stuff, you can't unlearn it. Once you understand what's really happening and that you have a choice, then it really is all up to you!

No more "But I have bad genes!"

No more "But I'm big boned!"

No more "But my life is really stressful right now, you just don't understand!"

Blah Blah Blah
No. More. Excuses.

You CAN lose weight with the Code Red Revolution.
You CAN keep it off by becoming a Rebel For Life!

Are you ready for this?
I'm with you all the way!

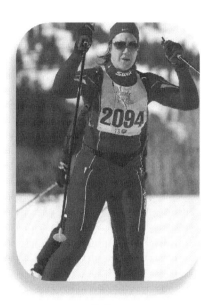
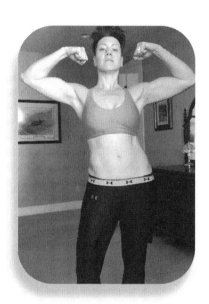

*Before*                                    *After*

━ ◄ CHAPTER 1 ► ━

# WHERE THE HEAD GOES, THE BODY GOES

**B**ECAUSE YOU'RE HOLDING this book in your hands, I'm guessing you've heard one of the following statements from a medical professional, fitness expert, or well-meaning friend or family member:

"You're just built this way."

"It's genetic."

"It runs in the family."

"You can't lose weight at your age."

"There's nothing you can do except take medication for your aches and pains and learn to live with it."

"If you can't exercise, you can't lose weight."

And because of lies like these, I'm guessing you've been circling the weight loss mountain for years, decades, or maybe even your entire life.

You've tried every diet you could get your hands on, no matter how *out there* it seemed.

You've tried every shake, every patch, every pill, and every powder.

You've spent hundreds a month on mail-order Frankenfood, and tried killing yourself in the gym for hours at a time.

Maybe you've even gone as far as weight loss surgery, because you truly believed it was your last hope.

Yet even after putting yourself through all that, none of it got you the lasting results you wanted, leading you to the inescapable conclusion that you're *destined to be fat.* Maybe you even believe that your body hates you.

Well I'm here to tell you this: you're not destined to be fat, and your body loves you.

**Destiny has nothing to do with it.**

I don't know you personally, but I'm guessing I have clients just like you. They've struggled to lose weight for a long time. Some of them tell us they've been heavy since childhood. They can't remember a time they weren't on a diet of some kind. Some of their past efforts were successful in the short term, but they couldn't manage to keep the weight off for good. All that failure weighs heavily on their hearts. They come to us in tears, desperate for a solution.

Their joints hurt. They're taking a long list of prescription medications to "manage" their health. They get winded walking up a short flight of stairs. They don't have the energy to play with their kids or grandkids. And some are afraid that if they don't get their weight under control now—they might not even survive the rest of the year. They are truly afraid they will die if they don't figure out the solution.

If any of that sounds like you, here's the first thing I want you to know: it doesn't matter what you've tried in the past, or how many times you've failed at weight loss.

It doesn't matter what genetics you've inherited, how long you've had a weight problem, how old you are, or how many kids you've had. It doesn't even matter what your family, friends, or even medical professionals have told you.

The reality is that there's nothing wrong with you, and that battling your weight is not your fate. In this book, I'm not only going to prove that to you, I'm going to reveal the TRUTH about why you have a weight problem. Then I'm going to reveal the simple tried-and-true solutions you need to put an end to your fight with your weight once and for all.

I know – a lot of "diet books" you've read make you that same promise.

That's why *Rebel For Life* is not a diet book. If anything, it's an ANTI-diet book, because the reality is that diets don't work. If they did, you wouldn't be reading this right now. I'm going to help you free yourself from the yo-yo diet cycle once and for all, by revealing all the things that keep you trapped.

We're going to make sure this is the last time you ever have to lose weight.

## WHY WE FAIL

You've been set up to fail and odds are you don't even realize it. There are very powerful industries out there that stand to lose a lot of money if you were to become aware of and embrace the truth about what it takes to live a long and healthy life, free of obesity, constant pain and disease. It's in their best interest to keep you fat, sick, and circling the weight loss mountain for as long as possible.

To make sure you stay stuck, they bombard you with the idea that one magical quick fix is all it takes. Just take this pill. Oh, wait, nevermind...try this shake instead. And when the latest gimmick or fad diet fails you—again—you're shamed into believing that it's your fault. Perhaps believing that it works for everyone *except you*, so there must be something wrong with you.

You're led to believe that it's YOUR fault you're fat. It's not because they're lying to you. It's because you're lazy. You lack willpower. You don't value your health enough to put down the donut and torture yourself in the gym. All that is bull crap, and by the time you're done reading this book, you'll understand why.

Sustainable weight loss cannot be accomplished with a magic bullet. I know that's hard to hear, but after 25-plus years in this industry coaching tens of thousands of people from all over the world, I can tell you this with absolute certainty.

Anyone who tells you that losing weight is easy is lying to you. You know it. I know it. They know it.

But it is achievable! You absolutely can lose all the weight you need to—whether that's 10 pounds or 210 pounds—you just need to keep your eyes on the prize.

It is simple – simpler than you've been led to believe.

## KEEP IT SIMPLE

On the opposite end of the spectrum from the unsustainable quick fixes are the complicated programs that overwhelm you with recipes full of weird ingredients you have to special order, and pages and pages of shopping lists. Who has the time or money for that?

You don't need to be a gourmet chef and spend hours in the kitchen to lose weight. Nor do you need to buy a bunch of expensive testing devices. You don't even need to worry about eating organic unless you want to. All you need are real food, water, sleep, and a few simple rules. You'll also need the right mindset to make this work with your daily life. Adopting the Rebel mindset is the key to your success.

## WHERE THE HEAD GOES, THE BODY GOES

I grew up poor in a small rural Idaho town and becoming a professional boxer wasn't even on my radar. My parents, two sisters, and I lived and worked on a farm, and my parents poured every spare cent we had into maintaining our property and caring for our livestock. If my sisters and I wanted to go to college—or even wanted fuel to drive someplace—we had to get a job and pay our own way. So that's what we did.

I've always loved movement and exercise, so I decided to study nursing and exercise physiology at the University of Memphis while working various jobs, including bartending, to earn whatever income I could. One day while I was working out and taking my first-ever boxing lesson, a boxing coach noticed me practicing, walked up to me, and asked, "How long have you been boxing?"

I glanced at the clock and replied, "Forty-four minutes."

He went on to tell me I was a natural—good enough that I could make a career out of boxing professionally. *Really?* I thought. *What a weird thing to say.* I wasn't interested and told him as much. That's when he said, "You can make money."

As a starving college student paying her own way, I have to say that got my attention. When he said it paid more than waitressing, I was all in. But before he'd take me on as a student, he had one condition: I had to audition. That meant allowing a male boxer to beat me up. If I could stand up afterwards, he'd coach me.

I agreed to the audition, and as promised, a male boxer pummeled the daylights out of me. Afterwards, bloody, bruised, and beaten, I forced myself up off the ground, my legs wobbling underneath me, until I was standing all the way up. It took all the strength I had left. It was enough. He agreed to train me.

One of the first things I learned while training to fight was a universal combat principle that says, "Where the head goes, the body goes," which means where your head goes, your body goes. Years later, when I began coaching people through weight loss, I realized that "where the head goes, the body goes" doesn't just apply to fighting. It's also true about mindset.

Like me, you've probably heard about the importance of mindset, but most of us grossly underestimate exactly how much power our minds have over our actions, including our efforts to lose weight.

See, when you battle your weight for a long time - even your entire life - you develop this identity as "someone with a weight problem." Your experience tells you that it's hard for you to lose weight and that you always gain it back.

This identity you've built for yourself can be deeply ingrained. And unless you're able to transition to a new identity as someone who lives a full, healthy life while easily staying at a healthy weight, your risk of gaining your weight back multiplies exponentially. That's true even if you diet yourself down to your goal. If you still see yourself as "someone with a weight problem," your subconscious mind is going to make sure that your body reflects that. You guessed it—you'll gain the weight back.

Your mind fights your body like me fighting the guy in my "audition." You get pummeled, and you get back up again. You get knocked down, and you get back up again. Over and over, until you get out of the ring and quit or decide to make a real change on the *inside.*

I wrote this book to beg you to get back up one more time. Stop beating yourself up. Stop fighting with yourself. Enough is enough!

What it all boils down to is that *you can't become or stay a slender, healthy person while still thinking and acting like a fat, sick person.* Where the head goes, the body goes. The foods, lifestyle choices, and mindsets you're about to learn are designed to encourage that identity shift, ensuring you never go around this mountain again.

## YOU CAN BE FREE

It is 100% possible to lose your weight, keep it off, and enjoy a full, healthy life without feeling deprived. I know because I've got thousands of Code Red Rebels who are doing it. They're doing it with kids and families. They're doing it while traveling and working odd hours. They're doing it with diabetes and heart disease. There's no reason you can't be among them.

Two-thirds of people living in the United States are overweight; over one-third of them are obese and 88% are metabolically sick. Disease rates are skyrocketing, and Americans are on more prescription medication than ever before. You don't know it yet, but you're about to embark on a journey of healing. You're going to become healthy from the inside out. Humans weren't designed to need artificial help just to live. Joint pain and failing bodies are not a natural consequence of aging. They are a natural consequence of eating empty, processed, chemical-laden crap. They are a natural consequence of not getting enough water and sleep to rejuvenate your body on a cellular level. They are a natural consequence of living in a stress-filled world.

I can't make any promises about what you'll experience as a Code Red Rebel. *Really, the law says I can't promise anything.* However, I have thousands of examples of real people just like you who are getting healthy when they thought they had given up. I've seen them do miraculous things when they set their mind and heart on a path that works. They ate real food. They got lots of sleep. They drank lots of water. They didn't exercise themselves to death. They were successful!

Before we get started, take a few minutes and think about what's weighing you down right now. Besides your extra pounds—what would you like to lose? What numbers would you like to see change? What prescriptions would you like to never buy again? Write them down. Then close your eyes and imagine for a moment. What would it feel like to be rid of those things?

- Imagine yourself tossing that CPAP machine in the trash.
- What would you do with all the extra money in your pocket once your doctor takes you off medication?
- What new activities have you always wanted to try, but were afraid to?
- What would it feel like to get through an entire day without pain?

Write it all out. Take as much time as you need. Don't skip this step. It's an important part of the process! Before you can begin a journey, you've got to know where you're going.

You're going to discover that my methods are different. They're scientifically proven. And the results that Code Red Lifestyle™ clients get are undeniable. Legally, I'm not allowed to guarantee anything, because I can't control how you use the information in this book. However, our custom program clients typically lose 10% of their body weight every month until they reach goal weight. That usually averages out to between half a pound and a pound gone every day! Best of all, they feel better than they have in years. They aren't hungry. They have tons of energy. And they know they can sustain the losses over the long term.

Does that sound unbelievable?

I get it. You've probably been told that losing more than one or two pounds per week is "unsafe." Bullcrap. It's completely safe.

It's not achieved by tricking your body chemistry. It's not achieved by punishing yourself with excessive exercise. It's achieved by lovingly feeding yourself real food, in the right proportions. It's achieved by getting lots of sleep and drinking lots of water...and it's achieved with the other tricks up my sleeve that you'll learn in this book.

When my Certified Coaches and I help people lose weight, it's with the understanding that it is the LAST TIME they will ever have to do it! It's the LAST TIME around the weight-loss mountain. That means they're going to have to adopt some new mindsets and embrace some new ideas about nutrition. It also means they're going to have to reject what the billion-dollar food and diet industries have been telling them for decades. Are you ready?

## THE CRITICAL MOMENT

When I was 18, I ran off with a guy.

Not long into this relationship, he began beating me up. The abuse was physical and emotional. You know, being one of the premiere female fighters in the world, I can take a beating. (Unfortunately, I didn't become a pro fighter until I was 23. Five years after this relationship.) In some ways, the bullcrap he used to say to me took longer to recover from than the physical abuse.

Each time it got worse, and more than once he threatened to kill me. One night, he beat me up worse than all the times before. I remember waking up on the floor, just lying there in my own blood. It was, without question, the lowest point in my life. It was my rock bottom.

I knew I had to find the courage to get myself up off that floor and out of town, or I was going to die. I was physically and emotionally beaten down. It would have been easier to just lie there. The act of pushing myself off the floor, out of the puddle of my own blood was, to this day, the hardest thing I have ever done.

Everyone will face a time in their life when they feel completely beaten down, and they won't know if they can push themselves up off that floor. You will have that moment—that critical moment where you have to make a decision: get up off the floor and find a new way or lie there and bleed.

Rock bottom is different for everyone, and whether you're physically bleeding or just spiritually broken, it's all hard. At Code Red, we work with people who've reached that critical moment with their weight. It's do or die. They can't keep going the way they've been going for years. They can't be heavy anymore. And they'll do whatever it takes—if someone would just tell them the truth about what works.

This is your critical moment. It's time to decide once and for all that you are going to lose the weight no matter what it takes. The Code Red Lifestyle™ is how you do it. It's hard pushing yourself off that floor. I've done it. My clients have done it. I know you can do it, too. It's worth the effort.

YOU ARE WORTH THE EFFORT.

Life often throws us curveballs. That's never going to change. Curveballs, challenges, obstacles...they all make you work harder. Holidays will come and go. Birthdays, weddings, vacations—none of them are an excuse to give up. Everybody makes mistakes. When our clients have a bad week, slip up, and eat something they're not supposed to, my Certified Coaches and I will call them on it...but we won't give up on them. We won't give up on you. We know you can do this. You are stronger than you know.

## I'VE GOT YOUR BACK

Everything you're about to read is based on over 25 years of working with all kinds of people. It's grounded in science, and it works, but I don't want you to take my word for it.

You've been fed so much bullcrap over the years from the diet industry and the fitness industry and the media. You've probably bought into lots of random weight-loss philosophies and been disappointed. I get it. Why should this be any different? Just because I'm saying you'll lose weight doesn't mean you will. And just because you lose weight doesn't mean you'll keep it off forever.

- Read the whole book. I've tried to make it as easy to read as possible with small, easy-to-digest portions.
- Pay special attention to the success stories. These are people just like you. They are parents and grandparents, people with high blood pressure and diabetes, people who thought they had no hope. They found a way to believe in themselves. They followed the rules and they were successful!
- After you've read the whole book, try it out. Not just for a little bit. Dive in wholeheartedly. Follow the Code Red Lifestyle™ Facebook page. Watch my YouTube videos. Listen to my Rebel Weight Loss and Lifestyle podcast.

So I'll make a deal with you, okay? If you do these things, I'll do everything I can to help you.

I want you to see for yourself that this works. I want you to finally understand that you can lose weight predictably, without being hungry, without pills or powders, without spending money on weird diet foods, and without exercise.

You can do it. I know you can.

Then, once you've seen for yourself how well it works, I want you to talk about it.

Share this book!

Tell your friends. Help your neighbors out. Get your family on board... but not in an obnoxious way. When people see how well you're doing, they're going to be curious. They may be skeptical that it will work for them (just like you may be right now). That's okay. Give them this book. I'll do the rest. We're in this together.

Do we have a deal?

Awesome. I know you can do this, so let's get started.

Barbie Miller
Potlatch, Idaho
Age 47
90 pounds in 8 months


As a kid, I was always sick and in the doctor's office. My chronic fatigue began in junior high. I suffered with aches and pains the doctors couldn't explain. I missed a lot of high school because I was sick so frequently. I only passed because I was a good student when I was there.

I was never happy with my weight, but I wasn't truly obese until my mid-20s. After having kids, my lifestyle choices finally caught up with me. With age, my weight and more stress, more aches and pains developed. My chronic fatigue worsened and I got sick easily and more often.

Nobody had answers for me, despite my efforts to find them. My health was so poor, I developed chronic pneumonia and bronchitis. My airways were so sensitive, I saw an allergy doctor, who diagnosed me with food sensitivities. I tried eliminating the foods he indicated, and while it helped with some of my digestive issues, the other problems remained.

He advised me to follow up with a primary care doctor, due to my rash and abnormal autoimmune lab results.

My primary care provider ridiculed the allergy doctor's findings, scoffed at and dismissed my personal concerns, and recommended counseling. She claimed I was simply an overworked, overly stressed mom.

I lost a lot of faith in traditional medicine after that, but I wasn't ready to give up. I found a new primary care provider who specialized in non-surgical bariatrics. She prescribed a medically supervised nutrition plan based on Whole 30, and referred me to a rheumatologist.

The rheumatologist diagnosed me with fibromyalgia, and suggested I reduce stress, get quality sleep, and perform non-impact exercise. I wasn't content with that diagnosis, especially since getting more sleep and reducing stress seemed unattainable. Plus it took me a year to lose 25 pounds.

I wasn't getting the results I thought I should for the amount of effort I put in.

Later, I discovered a great chiropractor with a naturopathic approach. Although some of his recommendations helped, my problems persisted. They told me to be patient.

"It took you a long time to get heavy, so it's going to take a long time to shed the weight," they said.

A local naturopath said it was my thyroid. I'd already tried thyroid medication, and it had only made things worse. She tried a new medication, and it helped, but not enough.

At this point, I'd been diagnosed with fibromyalgia, subclinical hypothyroidism, chronic fatigue, adrenal fatigue, insulin resistance, brain fog, and chronic respiratory illness. Anytime a bug came through the house, I'd be the first to get it and the last to get over it.

I remember thinking, *If I feel like this at 44 years old, how am I going to feel when I'm 70?*

My drive to find the solution waned. I'd found pieces that helped, but no complete solution.

My social life dwindled. I no longer enjoyed my hobbies. I had a poor quality of life—I had no energy and was sick all the time. A "successful" day for me was being able to drag myself out of bed, shower, and go to work.

One day, I saw a former classmate posting on Facebook about his experience with Code Red. I watched him shrink before my eyes and thought, *If he can do it raising teenagers and working full-time, there's no reason I can't do it.*

Another challenge was starting soon, but I'd just totaled my car and my fibromyalgia flared up. So I talked myself out of signing up.

Still, I was skeptical. I believed the program worked, but would it work for ME? I'd tried so many different things, I wasn't willing to invest my depleted physical and emotional energy into just anything. I felt like a special case—that nobody was as bad off as me.

Cristy's one-to-one program seemed like my best bet, but I doubted I'd get my husband's support to invest so much money. When I finally mentioned it to him, he said, "Well, Barb, if you want to do it, I think you should."

Then Cristy announced another 10 Pound Takedown challenge, and I thought, *Here's my chance to dip my toe in the water without a huge investment.* I signed up right away before I could talk myself out of it.

I sent a group message to my family. "I'm doing this. I want to do this and I have to do this. Does anybody want to join me?" Both my daughters, my mom, and our respective spouses joined in. My mom even talked my brothers and my sister-in-law into signing up.

I entered that challenge determined to win it. I started drinking water and getting mentally prepared, and once the challenge officially began, I went whole hog.

During detox, I experienced headaches, irritability, andI felt a bit more tired. But since I was fatigued all the time anyway, it wasn't a big deal. That only lasted a few days. Despite those detox symptoms, I was losing weight and feeling better in other ways.

The improvements I noticed made it easy to stick with Code Red and follow all the rules. I wanted to go further, so I had to decide whether to do a custom program with Cristy or choose the home-study version. In the end, I made the choice that felt the *least* comfortable to me—the one-on-one—because I knew it would challenge me more.

I learned that discipline, routine, accountability, and planning are all part of what makes Rebels successful. I knew I had to be out of bed and weighed by a certain time of day. I knew I had to log my food into my Lose It app by a certain time of day, and that I had to have my food intake for the day all planned out. Lack of planning, discipline, and commitment all contributed to my past failures.

During my one-to-one, I still faced some health issues. At one point, I gained five pounds in two days even though Cristy and I had everything dialed in. I feared the other shoe had finally dropped and that I was that special case Code Red couldn't help.

Cristy knew something else was up. Two days before, my thyroid medication dose had been increased. It affected more than my weight. I had skin issues and fatigue. All of it—including the five-pound weight gain—was because I no longer needed my thyroid medication.

I stopped taking it and dropped those five pounds in two days. Following the rules and getting everything dialed in allowed us to get right to the real problem.

The year I found Code Red was stressful, especially at work. Despite that, I followed the program. I didn't miss the food that I had to avoid. My family was supportive. They saw how I was changing—not just losing weight, but also feeling better. Many of them joined me, and they all felt better as they lost weight too.

After my one-to-one time with Cristy ended, I felt confident in my ability to continue. Between the small-group coaching environment and my family's support, I had the tools to be successful.

Throughout my adult life, I've kept weight logs. It was fascinating to go back through those logs and see my progress. Dropping below 200 pounds was exciting, but it hadn't felt that out of reach.

Hitting 155, on the other hand, was an incredible milestone, because it was the lowest recorded weight I could find. However, I didn't use hitting 155 as an excuse to cool my heels. I celebrated, but I knew I had more weight to lose.

As exciting as it was to lose weight, it was even more exciting to stop getting sick all the time. I'm now the healthiest I've ever been. Even when everyone else gets sick, I'm usually fine. If I do get sick, I get over it quickly.

I get out of bed every day pain-free. The chronic fatigue is gone along with my fibromyalgia symptoms. Stress still affects me physically, but it's not as bad as it used to be.

I've got so much energy! I'm no longer stuck on the sidelines of my own life, watching my husband and children enjoy activities I couldn't physically participate in. I've begun exploring what I'm passionate about. My husband and I are empty nesters now, and the world is our oyster!

I'm also losing what I call my fat-girl mentality, because the weight came off faster than my mental limitations.

My first summer out boating after Code Red, I remember gingerly stepping from one boat to the other, trying to conserve energy and minimize discomfort and risk of injury. Then I caught myself and thought, *What am I so worried about now?*

Being free of my mental limitations is just as exciting as freedom from the physical ones.

I'm not alone, either. Collectively, my immediate family members and I lost over 350 pounds. Countless others who were inspired by my story have signed up. Complete strangers have reached out to me. I love being able to pay it forward, because somebody once inspired me and that changed my life. I want others to have the same experience.

Connection with the Code Red community was critical for my success. I have faith that I can do this myself, but I also like knowing the community is there whenever I need it. We share recipes, successes, and struggles. Having those supportive, like-minded people around is invaluable.

When I first found Code Red, I didn't trust in myself. So I chose to trust in the program. I saw the results it could get, and I focused on that until I learned to trust myself again.

The Code Red Lifestyle is unlike all the other programs I tried. It's realistic. It's sustainable. The food is good, and the support is amazing. It's everything you need to take your life back.

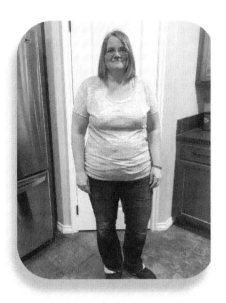
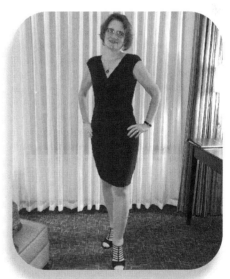

*Before*          *After*

---

◄— CHAPTER 2 —►

# WHY WE'RE ADDICTED TO DIETS

I T SEEMS LIKE every time you turn on the TV or hop on the internet, you see an advertisement for a new diet. If you're reading this, you've probably tried a lot of them. Every diet, pill, patch, shake, and gimmick – anything you can get your hands on. They all promise the same thing: Do almost nothing, eat what you want when you want, and lose all your weight.

I don't know what happened for you. Maybe the gimmicks sort of worked. Maybe they didn't work at all. Maybe you lost all the weight you wanted to, only to gain it all back with interest. Have you ever stopped and thought about why that keeps happening to you?

"Well, Cristy, it's because I didn't stick with it. It's my own fault. I just don't have any willpower."

Yes, it is true that in order for certain programs to work, you've got to follow them. But as a society, we're led to believe that not sticking with a "diet" is why diets fail. We're sold the idea that we're missing something, and that's why some of us can't lose weight and keep it off. This message is beaten into you left and right. Your willpower is the problem, not the "diet."

We're also shamed into believing that fat people are lazy, and don't care about themselves enough to make their health a priority. Once again the message is *it's your fault you're fat*. Even though I'm a big believer in personal responsibility, there's so much more to it than that.

As a weight loss expert and celebrity trainer who's been in the health and fitness industries for over 25 years, I've got decades of experience working with obese people. And I'm here to tell you—being obese isn't about being lazy. A weight problem is a symptom of some deeper problem—one that pills, points, and powders don't address. It's also a sign that your body is sick, and it's trying to protect you as best it can. Your body doesn't hate you, no matter what you might think. Your body loves you and is doing everything in its power to keep you alive.

Right now you're like a fly caught in a diet industry spiderweb, except you don't even realize you're trapped. Together, we're going to set you free.

## "YOU'RE WASTING OUR TIME"

One of my successful Code Red Rebels shared the most astonishing story with me about her past experience with a popular mainstream diet. She lost 35 pounds over a period of several months, and spent $150 a week on the company's processed diet foods. Then, once she lost her weight, she saw no reason to continue spending money on those foods, so she stopped. A representative with the company told her she was wasting the company's time, and to stop coming in for the weekly check-ins that were part of the program.

Pretty outrageous, right? It gets worse. Six months after kicking her out of the program, the company called her up about a special they were offering, because they knew she'd probably gained her weight back! They wanted her money and knew just how to get it. Diets will ALWAYS fail you because that's what they're designed to do.

## THE DIET MENTALITY

Most of my clients tell me that they've tried every diet under the sun. If they saw an ad or heard about it, no matter how crazy, they'd try it. We've all been conditioned from a very young age to accept the diet mentality. You're expected to make a temporary change to lose the weight, and then return to the same foods and habits that caused your weight (and health) problems in the first place.

It's like saying you only need to have an engine in your car the first time you want to drive it, but after that, no engine is required. When you say it like that, it sounds absolutely ridiculous, doesn't it? Yet we buy right into it, never stopping to question whether or not it makes sense.

It doesn't matter how smart we are, we all fall for it, and that's because our culture is steeped in the diet mentality, and it has been for generations. Our mothers dieted. Our aunts dieted. Our grandmothers dieted. Diets have been all the rage for so long, we've accepted them as *the way things are.*

The diet industry is happy to perpetuate this false belief by offering up a never-ending supply of magic pills, shakes, powders, patches, and dangerous, unsustainable crash diets. They'll sell us anything to stop us from taking a step back and asking, "Will doing this also help me keep the weight off and stay healthy for the rest of my life?"

Since a new fad diet comes out every time you turn around, there's no shortage of bullcrap floating around to keep the brainwashing firmly in place. Each time a new diet, pill, or other gimmick comes out, we leap to try it, cross our fingers, and hope this time will be different. How's that working out for ya?

## THE HOLLYWOOD SECRET

I spent years as a personal trainer in New York. I trained elite-level athletes, models, business tycoons, and celebrities. *Allure Magazine* even recognized me as one of New York's top trainers. Other national magazines often contacted me wanting to know the "Hollywood Secret" to weight loss. And you know what I told them?

There is no "Hollywood Secret."

Magazine reporters didn't appreciate my transparency, so I rarely got featured. I get it, though. Their job is to sell magazines, and without another bullcrap "secret" to reveal, sales will suffer.

I wasn't going to invent some "secret" just to be featured in a magazine.

The idea of an instant fix to all our problems is pretty alluring. No one is immune to that desire because our brains are wired for comfort.

Most of us have a lot going on in one day, and if we can make things a little easier on ourselves by getting what we want quickly, we'll take it. A lot of great inventions have come from our brain's desire for comfort—everything from washing machines to automobiles and cell phones. This desire for ease and comfort makes us susceptible to things that really aren't good for us, like unsustainable quick fixes. The diet industry takes full advantage of this saying, "Eat whatever you want, whenever you want, and still lose weight with _____."

I get that the idea of managing your food intake doesn't sound fun. But how much time and money have you wasted on quick fixes? How many crushing disappointments have you endured as a result? Repeating the same patterns that are failing you won't get you where you want to be.

Do you want to gag down some weight loss powder or nasty shake mix for the rest of your life?

How about pills, or processed "diet foods?" Do you want to keep buying them forever? Unmasking an unsustainable gimmick for what it is comes down to asking yourself this simple question:

Is what I have to do to lose the weight drastically different from what I have to do to keep it off?

If the answer is yes, then you've got an unsustainable gimmick on your hands.

Sustainable weight loss and physical well-being require embracing a new lifestyle, with new habits and new choices. Shake powders aren't a lifestyle. Counting points isn't a lifestyle. Wearing a patch isn't a lifestyle. You don't want to gag down shakes or buy expensive diet foods for life, but as soon as you stop buying their products, what happens? All the weight you lost piles back on.

It's a vicious cycle that keeps you stuck in an impossible loop of failure upon failure.

Each failure reinforces the lie that there's something wrong with YOU.

Eventually you reach a point where you can't take the disappointment anymore, and you give up. This is just how you're *meant to be,* except, it's *not* how you are meant to be.

The first step in healing yourself and your relationship with food is deciding to stop listening to the people who want you to stay fat and sick, and start listening to those who will show you how to take control of your weight and health, FOR LIFE.

## IT'S NOT JUST DIETS

There's more money in fat, sick people than there is in healthy people, which is why the diet industry is not the only industry with billions—even trillions—of dollars on the line. Americans spend exorbitant amounts of money every year on medical expenses to treat health conditions directly related to obesity and poor diet. There's a pill for every ill. Surgery and medication have their place, but they shouldn't be the go-to solution for every single thing that ails us, *especially* obesity.

And yet, they are, even though the truth is out there.

How much money would drug companies lose if you, and everyone else, realized how much influence proper nutrition truly has on your well-being? It's in their best interest to keep you popping pills.

The food industry is another culprit. You know all that tasty processed junk food you can eat and eat and eat, and never get enough of? The fact you're never satisfied is not your imagination. Food companies pay the most brilliant scientists and chemists in the world to chemically engineer addiction into your food.

Human taste buds are grown in a lab, and scientists experiment on them to see which chemical concoctions excite them the most. Then the winning chemicals are engineered into foods that taste amazing, but contain zero nutritional value. The more you eat, the more you want, just the way the industry planned it. If you suddenly started eating rich, delicious, filling, real food, and stopped craving their junk food, they'd be out of business.

They can't have that.

## THE MODERATION MYTH

Moderation is touted by the diet industry as a way to enjoy your *favorite foods* while you lose weight. Unfortunately, most of your *favorite foods* are contributing to your weight problem. The more of them you eat, even in moderation, the longer it takes to get the weight off. That means you could be losing weight for weeks, months, or even years longer than you would if you just avoided these foods.

Not only that, but a lot of those *favorite foods* are chemically addictive, especially if they contain sugar. *Almost everything processed contains sugar.* Studies show that sweet substances are eight times more addictive than heroin. Suggesting that you eat sugary foods in moderation is like telling an alcoholic who's trying to get sober to consume alcohol in moderation. It just doesn't work.

I get that the idea of eating junk food in moderation and still losing all your weight is appealing, but it's not reality. Do yourself a favor, be strong, and just avoid those foods altogether during weight loss mode.

Andrea Dell
Boise, Idaho
Age 40
Lost over 30 pounds

I grew up a skinny kid. My diet wasn't exceptionally healthy or unhealthy. It was the typical mix of home-cooked meals and desserts, soda, and junk food. In college, I slowly but surely packed on the infamous "Freshman 15" with fast food and soda. After graduation, I spent two months cycling and walking all over parts of Sweden and Switzerland, including long walks down the Swiss Alps.

I lost seven pounds over those two months. I was so much more active that I assumed the weight loss was the result of my days spent walking and biking. Exercise as the solution to a weight problem had already been drilled into my head in school. My experience in Europe cemented it.

Once back in the US, I quickly gained back the weight I had lost, plus more. Of course, I wasn't walking or biking five to seven hours a day, six days a week. Who has time for that?

Before long, I reached my all-time high, at 40 pounds overweight.

Still convinced exercise was the answer, I tried running. I tried walking up and down very steep roads. I purchased home-fitness DVDs for Pilates, martial arts, yoga, Beach Body programs, and many more. I bought a gym membership and went consistently several times a week for years, doing things like cardio kickboxing and CrossFit. Some of it I enjoyed, some I hated.

In 2012, thanks to all those years of consistent exercise, I was the fittest I'd ever been, yet also the fattest. I kept telling myself, "One of these days it's going to happen. All this exercise is going to melt my fat away, just like that summer in Europe."

That day never came. I endured years of guilt, shame, and frustration. Was I not exercising long enough, or hard enough? No matter how much more I did, my weight wouldn't budge.

Then, in May of 2012, my health took a serious turn. I woke up one morning with a swollen, painful stomach. I was familiar with how belly fat felt—this was something different. As weeks passed, my health deteriorated. I suffered terrible heartburn, horrific dizzy spells where I was barely able to stay on my feet. Searing back pain twisted me up so badly, I had to see my chiropractor. He'd adjust me, and within hours, my back would twist itself back to its starting position.

The scariest part was that my swollen stomach compressed my heart and lungs so my body would forget to breathe. I'd suddenly find myself gasping for breath with no idea why. My heart felt like it was stopping and then rapidly starting up again.

One night, I was sitting alone in my living room, doing my best to face the fact that I might be dying. That one of these days, my heart would just give out and I'd drop dead wherever I was.

I went to the hospital and explained my symptoms several times. They ran tests, and conducted EKGs on my heart, but with the exception of insulin resistance, everything came back *normal*. They prescribed meds for the heartburn. My diet came up briefly. One PA told me to eat every two hours, suggesting low-fat and lean meats.

I didn't care what those tests said. I knew something was wrong with me, and I knew heartburn medication was at best, a Band-Aid. I'd stopped exercising for weeks because I wasn't physically capable of it.

That's how terrible my health had become in less than three months.

In August of that year, my dad suggested I see a naturopath who'd helped him and my stepmom. Figuring I had nothing to lose, I did. This naturopath was the first person to emphasize nutrition—not only for weight loss, but for overall health.

Following his recommendations—which included eliminating sugar, wheat, and gluten—all my symptoms disappeared within a matter of weeks. I lost 15 pounds with no exercise. Unfortunately, my weight crept back up over the next few years. Even though I continued to avoid gluten, I resumed eating sugar—far less than before, but enough to gain weight.

Finally, in May of 2017—five years from the onset of my health scare—I discovered the Code Red Lifestyle™. At the time, I was working at the Orofino newspaper.

One day, I overheard a coworker discussing someone our reporter was going to interview—someone named Cristy "Code Red." I didn't think much of it until I heard that she graduated from Orofino High School in 1994. We had attended high school together.

Cristy's message—that weight loss is 100% nutrition and exercise doesn't help—resonated with me. People I knew were following her program and seeing incredible results. These were people I'd seen yo-yo diet and exercise for decades and now they were losing weight SO fast.

Convinced I had nothing to lose by trying, I registered for her 10 Pound Takedown Challenge. (After all, the price point was less than I'd spent on my latest set of fitness DVDs.) I went in with an open mind and surrendered to the process. My way wasn't working, and I'd seen the results Cristy's program got for people. I believed it could work for me too.

That challenge blew my mind. Cristy emphasized the importance of water intake and sleep so adamantly. Her mindset training was powerful. And her confidence won me over to seeing nutrition as the key to weight loss and health.

Other people in the challenge lost weight, and I was excited for them, but my weight stubbornly bounced up and down by about four pounds. I followed the rules, ate the right foods, drank my water, and did my best to get the recommended amount of sleep.

Clearly, something was missing.

When Cristy mentioned custom programs, I knew I wanted one. The customization excited me—cookie-cutter weight-loss attempts never brought me results.

It took me a few weeks to work up the courage to invest in myself—it was a lot of money. When my program arrived, I scrutinized it, following along with Cristy's instructional video. Then I went to work implementing it.

At first, I didn't love logging my food, but I was determined to give my custom program everything I had. I remained open to Cristy's process, and looking back, that mindset served me well.

My determination paid off—I dropped 6.6 pounds the first week! I'd never experienced anything close to those results before. I SAILED past the lowest weight I had ever been able to reach on my own.

During this time, I attended a few social gatherings, all of which had loads of food. At the first two, I didn't eat at all. At the third, I brought my own pre-logged, pre-measured food. Abstaining from what everyone else was eating wasn't easy; but indulging just wasn't an option. My mind was made up to stay on-plan no matter what.

Partway through my custom program, I experienced that middle stretch where the initial excitement had worn off and my goal still felt far away. My motivation wavered, but I didn't quit.

I lost a total of 28 pounds on my custom program and hit my goal weight in under two months—beating Cristy's projected date for me by a week and a half.

It was exhilarating!

Few moments in life have felt as triumphant as stepping on the scale that morning to see that I was a full pound below my goal weight of 135, for the first time in almost 18 years.

Maintenance is an incredible experience, and I'm so grateful that Cristy teaches how to maintain weight loss. Nobody else I know of teaches that. I still weigh myself daily and drink all my water. I focus on getting enough sleep and I don't let junk food in my house. I absolutely LOVE maintenance.

Staying connected to Code Red has played a huge role in my success. I'd never had that supportive accountability in any of my other weight-loss attempts. (Frankly, I didn't want it, because I was ashamed at the thought of failing.)

Reading other Rebels' posts, encouraging them, and feeding off Cristy's excitement and encouragement during weekly coaching videos kept me connected and inspired. My success with Code Red even gave me the confidence to start my own business. Before Code Red, I never dreamed I'd have the courage to do something that daring.

I can't express enough gratitude to Cristy for what she's done. She showed up every day, tirelessly and passionately, and spread Code Red's hope and healing to the world.

She believed in me when I couldn't believe in myself.

So if you're unsure about trying Code Red, and I could give you just one suggestion to ensure your success, it's this: Let go of everything you—and the people around you—believe about weight loss. Enter this lifestyle with an open mind and give it your all.

It's okay if you're scared. If you can't believe in yourself yet, believe in those of us who have been where you are and come out the other side.

Experience the life-transforming hope and healing we enjoy. Surrender to Cristy's process, believe in it. This will take you further than you ever thought possible.

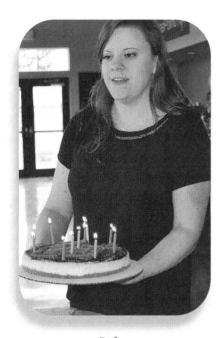

*Before*

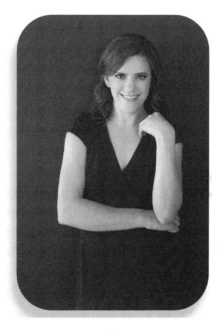

*After*

CHAPTER 3

# MEET YOUR CHEMICAL SURVIVAL SQUAD

YOUR BRAIN IS wired to keep you alive. That's job one. And it does that with loads of electro-chemical signals buzzing through your body every second. Unlike most mammals' brains, we learn many of our survival instincts through our personal experiences. That's why so many situations that aren't actually a threat to us still prompt a fight, flight, or freeze response, because when we were children wiring those circuits as we lived life, an angry look from mom *felt like* life or death.

Whether it's a bad hair day, a mugger waving a gun in your face, or your boss criticizing you, if you perceive a situation as a physical, emotional, or social threat, your brain is wired to release hormones that prompt you to respond in a certain way—a certain way that ensures your survival. For example, someone unfriending you on social media isn't actually a threat to you, but to your ancestors, social exclusion could literally mean death. Your primal brain doesn't understand that social media isn't the same as a critical family unit.

Sometimes there is no obvious immediate threat, just an uncomfortable feeling. Maybe you haven't been getting enough sleep or drinking enough water. Maybe you hate your job but aren't able to quit. You can't avoid uncomfortable feelings completely, so you naturally go seeking relief in the best way you know how—the way you learned as a child.

The good news is that since these responses are learned, they can be unlearned. Even better, you can teach your brain an entirely new way to respond to stressful situations. That means you don't have to be a slave to your brain chemicals. You have the power! Let's take a quick trip around your big beautiful brain so you see what's really going on when you unconsciously inhale a whole bag of chips.

When you're stressed or there's some threat to your survival, your body releases a chemical compound called cortisol. It warns you of potential threats and triggers your limbic system to be ready to take control and initiate a fight/flight/freeze response. When you have elevated cortisol levels, you feel like crap. Naturally, you will seek out ways to lower the cortisol so you feel better. Your body lowers cortisol with different *happy chemicals* designed to make you feel better—dopamine, oxytocin, serotonin, and endorphins.

These four happy chemicals each relieve certain types of discomfort. So it's important for you to recognize how to trigger the different types. Your body needs a healthy balance of all four to feel content. When you're content, cortisol stays low and your conscious mind is able to run the show instead of your cravings and habits.

## DOPAMINE

In addition to scanning for threats, the brain also scans for potential rewards. Dopamine is the signal you've found one. Long ago when humans were forced to hunt for survival, dopamine signaled a successful hunt, which meant the family got fed, which meant survival and continuation of the species.

Hunger (cortisol hit)—>Go hunting—>Take down a mammoth—>Dopamine hit—>go out hunting again the next time you feel hungry.

It's a habitual cycle that's hardwired into your survival system.

In short, it's an addiction.

Back to the doughnut example, if you're in the habit of using doughnuts to soothe emotional discomfort, when you see a box of doughnuts in the break room at work, dopamine gives you that "Woo hoo!" feeling.

Anytime you find evidence of something that felt good before, dopamine is what inspires you to go for it, even if it's destructive to you long-term, or even if it doesn't meet an actual survival need.

A text message from someone you love, recognition and praise from your boss, the sight of a food you enjoy - all of it can trigger dopamine.

Simply put, dopamine motivates you to get what you think you need, both in the moment and down the road. It's the "Yeah, I did it!" feeling, and also the "This gets me what I need! I've gotta get more!" feeling.

Getting on the scale and seeing a drop is another experience that triggers dopamine. You haven't accomplished your long-term goal yet, but dopamine's letting you know that you're making progress, and to keep doing what you're doing.

The day you reach your goal weight also triggers dopamine, because you've finally accomplished that goal.

But then you're done losing weight, and the hit of dopamine stops.

That's when you find yourself asking, "Now what?" What we don't want to happen is for you to gain some weight back just so you can lose it again and feel that dopamine hit from seeing the scale drop. Yet that is what you've trained your brain to do. So you've got to find other ways to release dopamine.

Your willpower will eventually wear out in the presence of so much dopamine. In fact, even just the *expectation* of a reward will release dopamine. So just SEEING goodies in the break room will give you a hit, hijack your conscious mind, and force you to go consume *just one*.

This is why you must stay away from the temptations! If there's no junk in your house, there's no expectation of reward, so there's no dopamine hijack. You stay on course. Simple. There's nothing wrong with you for wanting to eat dessert when it's placed in front of you. It's nature. It's how you're designed. But you can outsmart that instinct—by simply staying away from situations where you might get chemically hijacked.

One great way to release dopamine is to celebrate the little things. Celebration = Reward. Too often we wait until we accomplish a huge goal before we celebrate (if we celebrate at all), which deprives us of good feelings triggered by dopamine. Celebrate every ounce lost, every inch lost, every medication dropped, every ring that fits again (or that you can finally take off) - ALL of it.

Most people expend exorbitant amounts of time and energy on what they do wrong, or what didn't go well. I get it. I expect a lot from myself. I'm always pushing myself to be better and do more. Celebrating the small steps and the non-scale victories (NSVs) on your path triggers more dopamine than saving it all for one big outcome. The happier you feel as you walk your path, the more likely you'll be to stay on it.

Every day pick one thing you did that day that you're proud of, even if it was just to get out of bed this morning when what you wanted to do was hide under your blankets all day.

## SEROTONIN

Serotonin is related to social status. It's triggered when you feel important. It's also related to competition and winning. Gaining other people's respect promotes your survival. Serotonin is triggered when you feel important. Being a leader in some part of your life triggers serotonin - whether it's to your kids, in your group of friends, in your community, or in your business.

If your family and friends are supportive of your new lifestyle, you will get a boost of this chemical. You'll feel good and are more likely to stick with the program. On the other hand, if you're constantly harassed about your food choices or urged to stay up past your bedtime, you may be tempted to go along with the crowd just to make them happy and get that hit. Be careful who you spend your time with and how their reactions are actually affecting you.

Want to feel close to people *and* stick to your food plan? Hang out with like-minded people. Join a club that puts the focus on being healthy, and serotonin will work for you instead of against you.

## OXYTOCIN

This happy chemical is also related to feelings of closeness and trust with other people. In humans, oxytocin is thought to be released during hugging, touching, and orgasm in both genders. In the brain, oxytocin is involved in social recognition and bonding, and may be involved in the formation of trust between people and generosity.

You may want to bump up the oxytocin in your system by calling a close friend. Physical touch is also a great way to release oxytocin—something as simple as playing with your dog for a few minutes could stop you from binging on a bag of chips. (Or my favorite—get a massage!)

## ENDORPHINS

This happy chemical's core, survival-based purpose is to mask physical pain so you can escape harm. If you've ever fallen and gotten back up, only to discover a few hours later that your injury is a lot more serious and painful than you thought, it's because endorphins kicked in for a short time. A runner's high is a classic example of endorphin at work. Physical pain triggers it, but only for a short time, and only if you push past your capacity to the point of distress.

Obviously, inflicting more pain than you can bear on yourself so you can experience the euphoria of endorphins is not a practical or safe way to live, but there are plenty of safe, natural ways to trigger endorphins. Ever notice how good you feel after a big laugh? It's because laughing stimulates endorphins. Figure out what makes you laugh, and spend time doing it. "Fake it 'til you make it" does not apply here. It's gotta be genuine laughter. Find a comedian you like on YouTube, or spend more time with a funny friend. It's a great way to lower that cortisol.

Or you could try having a good cry. Yep! Crying, like laughing, is such physical exertion, your body releases endorphins in response. Crying often comes with some cortisol, so don't run around finding reasons to cry. Next time you feel the urge to cry, let it out. So many people stuff down the urge to cry, which creates unnecessary tension.

## STOPPING THE CYCLE

Every addiction or negative behavior started with a purpose.

No one says "Gee, it would be great if I could weigh 300 pounds and pay thousands of dollars for medication! If only I could have debilitating joint pain every day—that would be awesome!"

No, we end up in a bad place because of behaviors that were originally supposed to be helpful. We eat sugary cereal every morning because that's what our mom served us, and we love mom. We watch 4 hours of TV every night because it used to distract us from our parents' constant bickering. We avoid exercise because someone made fun of our shorts in gym class. All those behaviors are chemically driven.

Trigger—cortisol release—behavior.

Fight with spouse—cortisol release—ice cream.

It's automatic.

Great news folks—you can choose how you get your happy chemicals. And you can change your default behavior!

What's the solution? Wait it out. Sit with the discomfort. Acknowledge it. Listen for any messages it's trying to communicate.

By waiting and doing nothing when that uncomfortable feeling hits, you're giving your brain the space and opportunity to discover an alternate solution. If you're feeling bad, and your urge is to inhale three doughnuts, just wait. Give your brain time to make a different choice—a healthy, positive way to deal with that unpleasant feeling. Help your brain understand that just because you're uncomfortable does NOT mean you're about to die.

Your brain is smart, though. It takes milliseconds for you to go from a cortisol hit to inhaling a pizza. So you have to learn how to suspend time long enough to make a more rational choice. That is much easier said than done, so we're going to utilize a phrase you're most likely already familiar with—Stop, Drop & Roll.

Every time you feel a craving...

Every time you feel left out of the crowd...

Every time you're even tempted to break your promise to yourself...

Stop. Drop. And roll.

## STOP

Recognize when you're in a cortisol situation. Maybe your chest gets tight or you suddenly feel sick to your stomach. Whenever you feel triggered or stressed, train yourself to STOP whatever you're doing. Literally freeze in place whenever you're feeling discomfort.

This might take a while for you to recognize. You might be halfway through a candy bar. Or you may be able to catch yourself just *thinking* about eating the candy bar. It doesn't matter—just stop...take three deep breaths.

## DROP

Immediately drop into a state of suspended time. Pretend you're pushing a cosmic pause button that literally stops time long enough for you to think. Mentally step outside yourself and take an objective look at what's going on. Become an observer of yourself and try to figure out what's actually happening. You do this by asking yourself questions.

- What triggered the feeling?
- Was it real or imagined?
- Is your life actually in danger?
- Will giving in to your craving actually make things better, or will you regret it as soon as you polish off the last Oreo?
- What positive behavior could you engage in that would release happy chemicals into your system and relieve the cortisol?

## ROLL

Push the cosmic play button, return to real time, and roll on with whatever positive behavior you came up with. Take a walk, play with your dog, dance around the room to your favorite song...in a few minutes, you're going to make a whole list of possibilities.

Please do not think you have to wait until you've lost all your weight to use these strategies. Absolutely follow them in weight loss mode. The sooner you teach yourself that you don't need food to feel good, the more successful you'll be, both now and over the course of your life.

When cortisol rises to higher levels, you MUST relieve it. It's a survival instinct that is HARDWIRED. You have no choice but to seek out happy chemicals to handle the cortisol surge. It's how your body knows what behaviors to repeat in threatening situations. If you're sad/mad/bored...you will scan for the fastest, easiest chemical hit you can find. Also, the one that's habitual...the one that's never let you down before.

If a donut is present, and that's the only choice—you WILL eat the donut. Period.

If there's a CHOICE between the donut and, say, taking your dog for a walk or chatting with a friend or solving a crossword puzzle...well, then you have a little more control. IF the options are RIGHT THERE and you don't have to think too hard.

You have to put time between the stimulus (cortisol hit) and the response (dopamine hit). That's why you stop, drop, and roll. And that's why you need a go-to list of happy chemical-releasing activities to use instead of turning to food every time you feel uncomfortable.

## 100 WAYS TO FEEL GOOD

Getting pleasure and avoiding pain are the motivation behind every choice we make. Eating food brings most people a lot of pleasure, even if it's food that causes pain in the form of obesity, disease, and long-term emotional suffering. Food tastes good and it's readily available in most places. For this reason, most people have lost sight of the fact that food is not the only way to feel good. Not even close! There's SO much in this world that brings you pleasure, if you'd just think to look.

In fact, that's exactly what I'd like you to do.

Take out a couple sheets of paper, or open a blank document on your computer, and make a list of 100 things that make you happy. It's very important that nothing on this list of 100 is food-related. It can literally be anything. Petting your dog, using your favorite pen, hearing your kid giggle, reading a good book, listening to your favorite song, watching a sunrise...like I said, anything.

Once you've got that list of 100 non-food ways to feel good, pick 10 things that you can do anywhere, anytime. Put those 10 non-food ways to feel good somewhere you can easily access them. It can be on your phone, in your journal, in your car, or even taped to your bathroom mirror. When you feel the urge to eat in order to cope emotionally so that you can feel better, pull out that list and do at least one activity. Do this consistently, and you will train yourself out of sabotaging yourself with food.

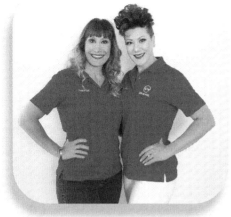

*Cari with Cristy*

Cari Thompson
Hardinsburg, KY
Age 46
Lost 110 pounds

I've never been a thin person. In high school, I hovered around a size 14 or 16 because I loved to eat! I always blamed my extra weight on being a "bigger girl" or having "big bones." I just figured that's how I was. It got to the point where 180 turned into 190, which turned into 200. A few bad relationships later and I was up to 260 pounds in what seemed like a heartbeat.

Weight gain happens insidiously. You don't even realize how big you've gotten until you turn around and you're 100 pounds overweight. Some people have horrible trauma and stress that causes them to gain weight. For me, it was just shoving too much food in my face. I fell for the low-fat, whole-grain lifestyle that society pushes on us.

When my kids were little, I remember going to Sonic and getting myself and the kids each a meal—a hamburger, fries, and a giant Coke. I would eat mine, but the kids would only eat a couple of bites. So I would eat theirs too. I would eat like 3,000 calories at a time without even realizing it—a great way to get fat. You don't notice it happening because you're just busy. I would eat mindlessly and then get on with whatever else I was doing.

I remember my turning point like it was yesterday. Years back, we took a family trip to a Six Flags in California. I love roller coasters, especially the old wooden ones. Our society today is pretty accommodating toward heavy people, but that wasn't always the case. Well, I climbed into one of the old-fashioned wooden roller coasters and I couldn't fasten the seatbelt. I stretched it across my lap and tried to click it in. No click.

Everyone was watching. I started sweating that nervous sweat that trickles down your neck. My hips were so big, I couldn't wear a roller coaster seat belt. To make matters worse, the poor kid running the ride came over and tried to assist me. He was laying across me, straining with all his might to click my seatbelt, to no avail.

I felt like this fat girl holding up the ride. The kid trying to help me was sweaty and his dreadlocks were in my face. My cheeks and chest flushed with embarrassment. It was utterly humiliating.

Ultimately, he gave up. That seatbelt would not click, so I had to climb back out and exit the ride. My son had to get out as well because he was too scared to ride by himself. I thought, *I can't even go on rides with my kids anymore.* And I felt this heavy, sick weight on my heart.

For years, I actively denied my weight. I avoided seeing myself in a full-length mirror. I would check myself from the waist up, just to make sure my hair and makeup were good. I kept buying bigger sizes, telling myself things like "I'm just a big-boned girl" or "Butts just run bigger in our family." Now, 110 pounds down, that mirror trick is one way I can tell that I'm starting to creep up again. If I catch myself not looking in full-length mirrors, I know something is off.

I made excuses for my behavior all the time. I was a nurse working 12-hour shifts—who has time for fitness? And in your 20s, you can compensate for a while. I could not have managed that workload at that weight if I had been older. I had health issues I ignored and made excuses for too. But I put it out of my mind...until that day when I couldn't go on a ride with my son. That was my turning point.

Initially, I turned to weight-loss surgery. Unfortunately, I had ALL sorts of complications. Years later I ended up having more surgeries to REVERSE the procedure and correct all the issues it caused!

I did lose a little weight in the beginning, but it failed to address the real problem—I was addicted to diet soda and sugar. That surgery cost me a lot of money and pain I could have avoided if I had just paid attention to my sister, Cristy.

Everybody has a turning point, and it doesn't have to be 110 pounds. Your turning point could be when your favorite jeans don't fit anymore, or you see a photo where you don't even recognize yourself anymore. You don't have to be obese before you have a turning point. It could be that you had a baby and are struggling to lose the pregnancy weight.

If you've tried countless shakes, diets, and pills, it is definitely your time. I used to spend money on thermogenics and take a pill three times a day, I was so desperate. That was not the right plan, and it was not the right time. My right time was when I couldn't ride a roller coaster with my son.

The biggest truth I had to face was that I was completely and helplessly addicted to sugar and diet soda. One of the biggest lies our society tells us is that diet drinks won't affect us the same way sugar does. Baloney! When I was drinking that stuff, I was hungry and thirsty all the time. And I tried everything to lose weight. I drank the shakes. I took the fen-phen. I went to all the weight-loss meetings.

Nothing worked until I listened to Cristy.

When I finally quit drinking diet soda, I felt like a junkie coming off narcotics. I work as a nurse in the intensive care unit and I see what it's like when people come off meth and heroin with the tremors and nausea and the headaches. It was that bad.

It's amazing the number of chemicals that leave your body when you start eating healthier. You really have to be prepared for that and decide that taking your life back is more important than ever drinking another diet soda or eating another piece of bread. It doesn't matter if you weigh 120 pounds and only want to lose 5, or you're 260 like I was and need to lose a heck of a lot more—the addiction is the same. I didn't start to heal until I faced the fact that diet soda and sugar were killing me.

Now I was lucky, because Cristy is my sister. So when I finally decided it was my time, she was right there to help me. But that doesn't mean I got off easy. I had to follow the rules the same way everyone else does. She got on my case every time I started to stray, even when I was in the hospital having surgery! Thank goodness the rules are simple.

I stopped drinking diet soda. I started drinking water. I ate real food. *I now weigh less than I did in high school.*

It's amazing to be able to buy the clothes that I want to wear and look at myself in a full-length mirror. Sometimes I'll catch a glimpse of my reflection in a window and think, "Who's that pretty girl?" Then I realize it's me! No matter how much or how little you need to lose, you can absolutely do it with Code Red.

It's so exciting when it's *your time.* And the best part is that since you get to decide when that is, it can be *right now!*

## 9-YEAR UPDATE

One of the biggest changes for me since I started the Code Red Lifestyle in 2011 is that I've developed a more balanced view of keeping my weight off. I know my weight will fluctuate, and I know that's okay, so long as it stays within the range I want it to.

I also began working for Code Red, and my family and I moved to a different location.

The gastric surgeries I had before Code Red, along with my lifestyle choices for years (including abusing food), have resulted in more significant and longer-lasting health complications. I now deal with chronic anemia and have to receive iron infusions every two to six months. I've had massive kidney stones. I need regular B12 injections and I'm monitored by a hematologist.

Like so many others, I went into weight-loss surgery believing I'd come through it unscathed. Some people do, but a lot of us end up with absorption and malnourishment problems for years afterward.

I will live with these complications forever, so please take it from me when I tell you there's no need to put yourself through this when the Code Red Lifestyle is available to you.

Accepting who I am and switching my focus from being thin to being fit and healthy has been key for my long-term success. Another thing that's been crucial is staying connected to the Code Red community and all the people in it who believe like I do.

Every bite I eat either makes me healthier or takes me further away from that, so I make a point to fill my mind with inspiration and consistently examine my eating habits. For example, I reread Cristy's first book, *The Code Red Revolution* and I listen to her podcast regularly.

It's so important to remain vigilant. Not to the point where you're miserable and constantly worrying about your weight, but enough so that you don't become complacent. Stay on the scale. Drink your water. Keep the junk out of your house.

When the little things start to slip, next thing you know you're pulling out the fat clothes and telling yourself, "Oh, I just want to be comfortable," when the reality is that your jeans no longer fit because you've gotten lax.

Stay mindful, stay accountable, and stay connected to people who believe what you believe.

---
CHAPTER 4
---

# THE REBEL FOR LIFE IDENTITY

I CAN TEACH YOU all about nutrition, water, and habits, but if your mindset and identity stay stuck where they are now, it won't matter. You'll lose the weight. You'll think you're good to go. You'll gain that weight right back. I've seen it over and over in two and a half decades in the health and fitness industries.

Think of it like giving a carpenter a hammer. This carpenter could be the best in the world, with the highest-quality hammer. But if they don't believe it'll work, it's useless.

It's the same with the Code Red Lifestyle. You have to believe it's going to work for you. We have to address the mindsets and identity shifts that will free you from the cycle of self-sabotage. I have to help you shift your belief systems so you can make the most of what you learn in this book.

Sound good? Then let's dive in.

## "I AM SOMEONE WITH A WEIGHT PROBLEM."

If you're like most overweight people I talk to, that's probably how you think of yourself right now. You may have held that identity most of your life. If so, it's completely understandable. Depending on how many times you've struggled to lose your weight and keep it off, you have years (or decades) of evidence to support your identity as someone with a weight problem. It's no wonder you've accepted it as your reality.

Your identity as "someone with a weight problem" is only your reality because you *believe* it is. When you see yourself in this way, it shapes your beliefs about what you're capable of. I've had clients whose identity as "someone with a weight problem" is so deeply ingrained, they lose all their weight and then sabotage themselves into gaining some back, just so they fit back into that identity.

The same thing happens with people who live their whole lives with the identity of "someone who's always broke" and then they hit it big in Vegas or win the lottery. They will spend all that money down to the level of their identity, so they can "be who they are" once again. No one wins the lottery and says, "Hey, you know what would be great? Let's blow all this money so we can live on ramen noodles again!"

No one ever said, "Woohoo! I reached my goal weight. I feel great. I love my new body. Now let's pack on 20 pounds so I can get back to normal." Yet it happens all the time.

It's subconscious and it's sneaky. You can't beat your brain. You've got to work *with* it instead. So, starting right now, we're going to start shifting you away from thinking of yourself as someone with a weight problem.

I'm not talking about lying to yourself. I get that when you look in the mirror, you see someone with a weight problem. What I want is for you to start thinking of yourself as someone who "lives a full, happy, healthy life." And yes, of course you'll be at a healthy weight as part of that healthy life. That goes without saying. Start adopting that identity, *really believe it*, and your brain will happily help you reach that identity. This journey is about you as a whole person, not just the number you see when you step on a scale.

You're becoming a born-again Rebel, which means that old identity has got to go, along with the parts of it that aren't serving you – the habits that you have, your beliefs about yourself and about food, your self-criticism, your negative self-talk. All those things contribute to your weight problem.

Think of your life like a long forest path, full of dips and hills and twists and turns. Except on this path, you get to decide when and where the turns happen. Diets are just detours. They take you on a little side trip, but you end up right back on that same stretch of path where you're miserable.

The Code Red Lifestyle, on the other hand, is like turning onto an entirely new road that leads to a different destination. If the road you're on is leading you to a future full of pain and suffering, you can choose a different way. In order to keep you headed in that new direction, instead of turning around and getting back onto that old road, your old identity as someone with a weight problem has to go. So how do you make this shift? By adopting some new truths.

## THE NEXT STEP VS. THE END

The very first thing we need to address is the idea that there is an end to your path. So much of our world conditions us to expect a final destination. Books, movies, and TV shows all have an end. Our childhoods end. There's an end to high school and college. Sometimes our relationships end, or our jobs end. We're programmed to expect some kind of ending, and the diet mentality feeds right into this expectation.

Remember the definition of a diet: Believing you can make a temporary change to lose the weight, and then return to the habits, mindsets, and food choices that caused your weight gain in the first place. In other words, when the diet ends, you're conditioned to believe you get to return to what you were doing.

Except it doesn't work like that.

We can get so fixated on the end of something that when we finally get there, our subconscious mind asks, "Now what?" Life doesn't stop just because you reach a goal. Outcomes are just checkpoints on the path of your life. They're not the end of the path.

All those times when you finally got the job, finally got the relationship, finally got the money, finally had the baby, didn't stop your life from continuing, right? It is the same with losing your weight. Reaching your goal weight isn't the finish line. The day you get there is a great day, but it's still just a checkpoint.

It's really important to begin this mindset shift now, because when you follow the Code Red Lifestyle, you're *going to lose the weight*.

Once you reach your goal, you don't want to fall prey to "now what?"

syndrome and start backsliding just because you haven't given any thought to what's next.

What's next is that you continue on the path that is your life. Except now you get to do it following a lifestyle that promotes health and happiness.

## WEIGHT LOSS IS A TOOL, NOT A LIFESTYLE

If what you do to lose your weight is drastically different from what you do to keep it off, that's a huge red flag. It means you're dealing with something that's unsustainable for the rest of your life.

Code Red Rebels eat real food, drink water and sleep, both to lose the weight and to keep it off.

During the initial weight-loss mode, you will be more focused. You'll follow the rules to the letter. Then some rules and habits will continue after you've reached your goal and some won't. You will always have weight-loss mode as a tool in your toolbelt, to pull out any time you need it, but weight-loss mode is not meant to be a way of life. Real food, water and sleep, are what will become your way of life—forever.

## A NEW KIND OF FOOD FREEDOM

When you read the words "food freedom" you might think *Yippee! I can eat what I want, when I want, as much as I want!* That's not my definition of food freedom. See, in our world today, we are hyper-focused on food. We whip it out for just about any reason. Whether it's snacks at the office, the holidays, a birthday party, or a ladies' game night, we make it revolve around food. It doesn't matter what's going on—there's always a reason to overindulge.

Celebrating a new job? Great! Let's go out to eat.

Commiserating after losing a job? Oh no! Let's binge on junk to help us feel better.

Taking a trip? Cool! How many different restaurants can we hit?

If you think I'm exaggerating, recall the last special occasion you attended. Was there food present? Did you, and everyone else, eat a lot of it?

Can you imagine attending that special occasion without food being present? I bet the answer is *no*, or at the very least, *I don't know.*

It's fine if food is a part of gatherings or special occasions. I'm not telling you to starve! But what you eat does not have to be front and center in everything you do. There are countless other ways to enjoy trips and spend time with friends and family. Play a game, do a puzzle, go on a walk, or just enjoy each other's company.

When I bring this topic up with clients who are still hyper-focused on food, they'll sometimes say things like...

"Are you saying I can't eat foods I enjoy?"

"Are you saying it's bad if I enjoy cooking?"

Not at all! What I'm saying is that our world's food obsession is over the top. It's all most people think about. It's not healthy—mentally or physically. Food freedom means embracing the idea that not everything in your life has to revolve around what and when you eat. Adopting that mindset will go a long way toward establishing your new identity.

Ignoring food completely can be equally obsessive and unhealthy, especially if you're prone to severe restriction followed by binging. There's so much more to life than what you eat and when you eat. When you accept this, it will set you free.

## EMPOWERED, NOT DEPRIVED

*I just want to lose weight without feeling deprived!*

That's a thought you've probably had more than a few times while trying to lose weight. I get it. We wanna be able to eat what we want, when we want, and still look and feel healthy. The problem is, the food we think we want - because it tastes good, or we have emotional attachments to it - isn't going to help us look or feel healthy. Exactly the opposite is true!

Someone who wants to drink half a case of soda a day and eat a pizza for dinner every night is depriving themselves of being able to fit comfortably into their clothing. That sweet tooth is depriving them of getting on an airplane without asking for a seatbelt extender. That bottle of wine with dinner every night is depriving them of playing with their grandkids. See where I'm going with this? By choosing inflammatory junk food over your health, you're depriving yourself in other ways.

- You're depriving yourself of how it feels to look in the mirror and see something you love.
- You're depriving yourself of how it feels to go an entire day without enduring constant pain.
- You're depriving yourself of the physical and mental stamina to enjoy your favorite activities.

The deprivation mindset is rampant in the diet mentality. It says, "I'll deprive myself of the foods I love just long enough to lose some weight, then go right back to eating what I want when I want."

Do you understand how that sets you up for an endless cycle of failure? Part of living a healthy, happy life is accepting that you are worthy. You are worthy of love. You are worthy of enjoying life. You are worthy of good, clean fuel for your body.

Yes, it's going to mean making different choices with your food. It also means you get to feel amazing! You get to feel proud of yourself, and live a life free from obsessing over a weight problem that you feel helpless to do anything about.

Here's the best part. As you'll soon see, the foods we eat on Code Red are so delicious, rich, and filling, you're not going to feel deprived eating them. Stale, limp salads with one tomato and one crouton aren't a part of this lifestyle. Yes, there will be some foods you avoid, but you're not depriving yourself of them. You are CHOOSING to avoid those foods because you are choosing something better for yourself.

## LISTEN TO YOUR BODY

In today's world we eat for every reason you can imagine. We eat as part of celebrations, gatherings with friends and family, and vacations. We eat because we were taught to clean our plate, or because it's meal time and that's just what you do. We eat because we're bored, because we're tired, or because it's simply a habit to plop down in front of the TV with a bag of microwave popcorn.

There are a million and one reasons we eat. Almost none of them have anything to do with being hungry. Think about it. Can you remember the last time you ate only because you felt hungry?

Do you even remember the last time you experienced the sensation of hunger?

You're going to learn to listen to your body. Because whether or not you're aware of it, your body is constantly sending you messages. It wants you to know when it's tired, when it's hurting, when it feels great, and also when it's ready for more nourishment.

Most people today are incredibly out of touch with the messages their bodies are trying to send them, including whether or not it's time for more food and water. Listening to your body is essential in order to transition away from being "someone with a weight problem."

Feed your body only when it needs fuel, even if that means keeping unconventional meal times, or skipping a meal once in a while because you're simply not hungry. Your body wants to help you. That's what it's designed to do...but you have to pay attention to the signals it's sending you. You'll be amazed at what you can hear when you start listening, including what your body needs to lose the weight, to keep it off, and to be an ally not the enemy.

## THE POWER OF HABIT

I've probably never met you, but I can pretty much guarantee that your habits are a factor in your identity as someone with a weight problem. You may have a habit of going through the drive-thru after work, or ordering an extra-large popcorn and 64-ounce soda at the movies. Smoking, drinking too much, or stopping by Dairy Queen twice a week—they're all habits. By definition, that means they are unconscious actions.

It takes far less energy to simply run a habitual routine over and over again than it does to make the individual decisions. Your brain actually stops thinking (to some extent) when you repeat a habitual action because it's saving energy. It doesn't need to consciously decide if you want that second scoop of Ben & Jerry's. Of course you do! You *always* choose double scoops. So why would this time be any different? Have you ever found yourself halfway through a bag of chips and thought to yourself, *wait, what am I doing?*

Humans are habitual beings. When people realize they have an unhealthy habit, they think they can just stop it, but that usually doesn't work because you're already finished by the time you realize you're repeating the habitual action. Believe it or not, this is actually the most efficient way to live. Imagine if our brains were not wired this way. We'd never get anything done! We'd constantly be re-learning the same simple tasks and making the same basic decisions every single moment of every day.

One of my habits is having afternoon coffee. For years, around 3pm I would take out the French press and make myself a treat. There is nothing especially bad about coffee. In moderation, it can give you a healthy level of caffeine. The problem with my habit wasn't the coffee. It was the whipping cream I put in it. For my body, having cream in my coffee twice a day was too much dairy. I wanted to be leaner and the calories in that whipping cream were taking up too much of my daily allowance.

So I took a look at the real reason I drank coffee in the afternoon and discovered I just really liked that hot, comforting drink. It wasn't the coffee, it was the relaxing break in the middle of my day. Then I realized I didn't need to drink coffee. I could replace that habit with a different one.

So I switched to tea. I bought myself a cute little teacup and saucer, and a pretty teapot to match. Both made me feel good. I don't put cream in my tea, but the preparation is similar to the French-pressed coffee. To my brain, it feels pretty much the same. At the same time every afternoon, I set a pot of water to boil and I have my hot drink. All I did was replace the coffee and cream with tea and a pinch of stevia. My habit is still to have a hot drink every afternoon, I just switched what that drink was.

Creating new habits that support your new identity without shocking your system is an important part of your identity shift. If I had tried to just give up my afternoon ritual cold turkey, it wouldn't have lasted very long.

If you have a habit that you want to change, try replacing it with a different habit. Maybe your family enjoys ice cream every Sunday, and your weight is creeping up. Can you replace the ice cream with a small bowl of berries? Or could you send them out to get their ice cream while you stay home to enjoy a few minutes of blissful quiet?

Instead of sitting down in front of the TV with a bag of chips, create a habit where you sip a cup of tea instead. Or keep your hands busy with a craft project or fidget toy while you're enjoying your favorite show. Either way, stick with it, and soon it will become a new habit.

I don't want you to think I'm making light of habitual behavior. I know it can be difficult to make changes, especially when other people are involved. To help you form habits that support your new identity, I highly recommend reading *The Power of Habit* by Charles Duhigg and *Atomic Habits* by James Clear. These books will change your whole understanding of why we do what we do out of habit and how to make the necessary changes.

Be mindful of your habitual thoughts too. When you catch one that's not serving you, replace it with one that does, just like you do with your physical habits. If you catch yourself thinking, "I'll never get this weight off," switch it to "I am following this new lifestyle to the best of my ability, and I can't help but lose all my weight and keep it off."

Your habits can work for you or against you. Your choice.

Cassie Adams
Orofino, ID
Age 44
Lost 75 pounds in 4 months

My struggle with my weight didn't start until adulthood. I married my husband, Tim, straight out of high school. We lived in a fifth-wheel trailer, traveling from place to place for Tim's work as a helicopter mechanic.

Tim was eight years older than me and still awash in the "single guy mentality." So after work, or on weekends, he'd head to the bar with his buddies. I was under 21 and couldn't join him, so I was stuck alone in the fifth wheel, completely cut off from my family and friends. I felt so isolated and alone, so I began soothing my depression with food. That's when the pounds started piling on.

A break from helicopter life took us back to my hometown, where my difficult pregnancy with our first child ended in an emergency C-section. While there, we tried starting a gym, but it didn't work out and we had to file for bankruptcy. Six weeks later, we learned I was pregnant with our second child.

We had no money and no jobs, plus a one-year-old to provide for. So we decided Tim should reenlist in the army. They shipped us to Texas, where our second daughter was born. Once again I found myself far away from family and friends, this time with two small children to care for.

We moved again, had our third child, and after Tim served in and returned from Korea, we decided to have a fourth child. Shortly after Andrew was born, the doctors told us he had a heart murmur. While there was nothing wrong with his heart itself, everything that connected his heart to his lungs was too small for his body.

One early February morning that year, we drove Andrew to Sacred Heart Children's Hospital in Spokane, Washington, for a procedure. When it was done, medical staff woke Andrew so he could eat. We watched a nurse disconnect tubes and wires from Andrew right before she woke him up, but when she plugged Andrew's heart monitor back in, it showed that his heart had stopped. Doctors and nurses scrambled, life-saving medicines were within easy reach.

Andrew was gone.

Within six months of losing him, we also lost my 12-year-old nephew and a 20-year-old cousin. My world was completely shattered, and I still had three kids to take care of. Since I couldn't fall apart, I turned to food.

It was a relief when Tim received orders to head to New York. I couldn't wait to put some distance between us and the town where we suffered all those horrible losses, but as soon as we arrived in New York, Tim was deployed to Afghanistan.

While he was overseas, I enrolled in Weight Watchers to give myself something positive to do instead of just eat. I got my weight down to the 150s, but then I stalled, and no one in Weight Watchers could tell me what I was doing wrong. The little old lady who ran our local group told me, "Well, that must be all you're going to lose."

When Tim returned, he was SO proud of me. But since I'd enrolled in Weight Watchers because he was away, I had no reason to stick with it once he returned, and my weight soared back up.

Cristy and I went to high school together, and we reconnected on Facebook while I was living in New York, where she was living as a personal trainer. I watched as she moved to Boise and created the Code Red Lifestyle™. I was intrigued by the one-on-one nutrition and weight-loss coaching she offered, but it was out of the question for me. I still lived in New York and couldn't meet with Cristy in her Boise office.

After that, Tim got a job and we moved our family to southern California where we lived for two years. It was a really rough time in our lives. Tim struggled with PTSD from his deployment.

I reached the heaviest I'd ever been at that point. I was wearing size 16, 18, sometimes size 20 pants. It was the worst I'd ever felt.

After that, we returned to my hometown. Our marriage and our lives were in shambles. I was in such a dark place that I was ready to throw it all away.

Thankfully, I happened to be on Facebook and saw that Cristy was offering a weight-loss challenge called the 10 Pound Takedown. It was only $37, so I signed up.

I learned what to eat and what not to eat. I learned Cristy's Top 10 Rules For Consistent Weight Loss. I had everything I needed to finally succeed.

Instead, I failed. Miserably.

It was my own fault. Instead of trusting Cristy and trusting the results I was seeing in others, I caved to the little voice in my head—the same one that had sabotaged me my entire life.

Maybe I needed to fall on my face one more time, because failing at the challenge flipped a switch. I evicted that little voice, and even though money was still tight, I scraped up enough for a custom program.

The goal weight Cristy assigned me was less than I had weighed in high school, and no one but Cristy thought I could get there. People told me things like, "Being heavy runs in the family," and "You've had four kids, so your hips have spread."

I didn't care what they thought. When my custom program arrived, I decided I'd work it better than anyone ever had. My weight MELTED off. My clothing sizes dropped faster than I could shop.

When I bought the program, I didn't tell Tim, but it wasn't long before he noticed the difference. Finally he asked me what was going on and I told him what I'd done.

He had seen me try and fail at weight loss countless times throughout our life together, so he was pretty skeptical about Code Red. But as my weight kept dropping and I wasn't quitting, the last of his skepticism evaporated.

Four months went by and then came the day I'd been waiting for. When I stepped on the scale and saw that my weight had dropped BELOW my goal I'm pretty sure I woke up my entire house. I told everyone I could think of—my parents, coworkers, friends, and of course, Cristy, who was super proud of me. Tim was ecstatic too.

One thing that had sabotaged my past weight-loss attempts had been lack of a simple, realistic maintenance plan. Weight Watchers was the only program with anything like that, but it wasn't for me. I didn't want to count points for the rest of my life.

Cristy's program, on the other hand, includes an incredibly simple maintenance plan that doesn't require counting or tracking anything, while allowing occasional indulgences. I can have anything I want, and as soon as I eat it, I know what the scale is going to do. If it goes up, I know how to fix it.

When I started with Code Red, I was on daily blood pressure medication. Three weeks into my program, I stopped needing it. My grocery bill dropped to a fraction of what it had been, because the food my family and I ate was so filling. We just ate less (including my son, who was 16 at the time and had an impressive appetite.)

Going camping, traveling—everything costs less now and comes with far less stress because our lives don't revolve around when and where we eat next.

Even my marriage improved. I agreed to counseling—something I would not have done prior to Code Red—to try and save a marriage that was pretty much at its end. We did it—we saved our marriage.

**It was like my weight had become a shell, and losing it peeled back the layers to reveal everything I'd been hiding from.** I had to move forward. To do that, I had to reinvent myself and every aspect of my life. My marriage, my kids—everything.

A lifestyle change isn't easy and you've got to be ready. Otherwise, you'll just come up with a million excuses. Cristy likes to say, "Pick your hard, because it's all hard." That's how I knew I was ready. My "hards" were just too much. Being heavy was hard. Waking up every morning in pain was hard. The embarrassment of seeing that look on your kids' faces when you walk into their school and their friends see you was hard.

I spent 20 years trying to exercise my weight off. I owned more gym equipment than some gyms. I tried diet after diet. If I saw some skinny little thing promoting it, I bought it. So I know what it feels like to think that no matter what you do, it's not going to work.

Even though I had attended high school with Cristy, I struggled to trust her at first, and I paid the price by failing at the 10 Pound Takedown. That failure taught me an invaluable lesson. If I really knew best, I wouldn't have been fat in the first place.

If you're looking for proof that it works, it's there in all the success stories. Pictures are awesome, but the STORIES drive it home. Getting into the Code Red groups and talking to people who have lost it and kept it off, the trials and tribulations they have been through—there is no better proof.

If you can't trust yourself yet, trust all of us who have been there. Have faith that Cristy's program will work. The only thing you have to lose is weight...and for once in your life, *put yourself first.*

You might think that by spending time on or investing in yourself, you're taking away from others.

You're not.

*You're giving to yourself.* Therefore you have so much left to give to everybody else. When you don't give to yourself, pretty soon you won't have anything left.

I know this, because after 20 years of putting everyone else first, there wasn't much left of me to give anyone.

Choose you.

Choose a you that's moving forward to become someone brimming with energy—someone who wakes up pain-free in the morning—someone excited to see yourself in the mirror.

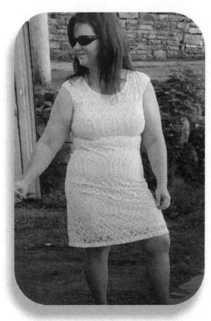

*Before*

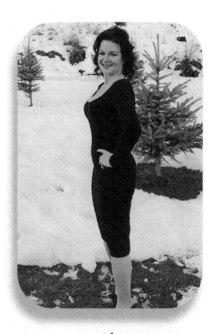

*After*

# CHAPTER 5

# STRATEGIES TO SUPPORT YOUR IDENTITY SHIFT

I T'S ONE THING to understand that you need an identity shift, it's quite another to actually achieve it! You might be thinking, *That's great, Cristy, but HOW do I do it?*

Here are 10 strategies you can use to start shifting your identity away from someone with a weight problem to someone who lives a full, happy, healthy life. Use as many or as few as you want, but pick at least one. Choose the one that resonates with you or feels like it's going to be most effective for you. By most effective, I don't necessarily mean easy; I mean the one that's going to actually work.

Right now you may not be sure which one it is, and that's okay. Choose the one that speaks to you and go from there.

## STRATEGY #1: USE YOUR WORDS

Scales are great and measuring spoons are powerful, but I'm about to show you the most amazing tool you have in your arsenal to meet any goal, especially weight loss: your own words.

Throughout this entire process, I want you to remember that this is all about you. You may have plenty of titles—spouse, mother, manager, sibling, whatever. But through this process, you have to focus on your health.

Everything else will fall into place once you are taking better care of yourself, but you must understand the power of your words.

The power of the words you speak is very real. For example, if you go around telling everyone that you have high blood pressure, you are more likely to continue to have high blood pressure. The more energy you expend on that subject, the more real it is.

I know it may sound a little "out there," but your words really do have the power to help or hinder you. If you constantly tell yourself that you can't do something, eventually that will be true, and you will have made it so.

I used to believe that I was not especially creative. I used to go around saying that to people. I would say that I wasn't an idea person, I was a follow-through person. Finally someone called me on it. "Stop saying that, Cristy—it's not true." And I stopped to think. I paint, don't I? I *am* creative, and I do have ideas. So why was I attacking my creativity?

We all struggle with negative, self-sabotaging thoughts sometimes. When that happens, just zip those lips. Ignore the thoughts and don't speak them out, because when you do, you're feeding that negative idea. Starve the negative ideas, and feed the good ones instead. Understanding the power of your words means being aware of your thoughts and only allowing the ones you want to become words. The thing is, as soon as you speak words aloud, you are giving them power. If you're going to give words power, make them good words like "I can do this." Yes, you can!

For those of you who are parents, you wouldn't let your kids put themselves down, would you? Don't put yourself down either! Think about what you are saying to or about yourself. If you wouldn't say it to a loved one, then you shouldn't say it to yourself.

This is part of healing yourself and taking your life back. You are being good to your body by feeding it healthy, nutritious food. Be good to your mind too, and don't put yourself down, okay?

You know the old saying "If you don't have something nice to say, don't say anything at all?" That is a rule I want you to abide by with yourself. If you can't find something positive to say about yourself, at the very least don't say anything negative.

We all have challenges in life. I am not asking you to ignore your problems, I am asking that you don't feed your problems by giving them a voice. The power of your unconscious mind is incredible and you need to make sure it is on your side.

When I wake up, I stand in front of my mirror and say, "You are strong, you are beautiful, you are healthy, you are smart, you are creative." I say those words out loud. I thank God out loud for strong legs when I am running. I say thank you for my back not hurting like it did when I ate unhealthy food.

Focus on the positive in your life. Those are the words you need to give power and life to. You can tell yourself what you need to hear. You know you need to cut out the junk food; it's time to cut out the junk words. Give your body nutritious food, and give yourself wholesome words and encouragement.

## I CAN, BUT I DON'T WANT TO

Years ago I attended a two-day conference where one of the treats they served was Rice Krispie treats. Let me tell you, I love Rice Krispie bars! I really do. But at this particular conference, I didn't have any. There was no willpower involved. I just didn't want them.

People ask me questions about my program all the time, and one of the ones I hear most often is "When can I eat the foods I want? When can I cheat? You know, when can I have the pizza and ice cream? When can I have the Rice Krispie bars?"

The first thing I try to clarify is what exactly they are asking. If they are asking when they can "cheat," the answer is *it depends on their goals*. Are they in weight-loss mode? If so, they avoid the ice cream or the pizza or whatever, until they reach their goal weight. If they are already at their goal and just trying to maintain and live a healthy lifestyle, then I guess they can have those things occasionally.

They are missing the point.

When you eat real food, without all the added sugar and chemicals, your mind switches to where you don't want that crap anymore. If you suffer from cravings all the time, I'm sure you don't believe me, but it's the truth. I didn't turn down the Rice Krispie bar because I had to or because everybody was watching. I didn't eat it because I didn't want to.

I didn't want to.

I finally got myself to the point where I wasn't craving it. I wasn't thinking about it at all. It wasn't an agonizing decision. It was a total *non-issue*.

That's what I want for you.

I want you to get to the point where you can, but you just don't want to.

Do I eat foods that aren't great for me? Yes, once in a great while, like when my husband, Miles, and I go out for our birthday or anniversary dinner.

You know what? It physically hurts me when I eat crap. It hurts my tummy. My back hurts.

It's a slippery slope when I eat carbs and sugar. It makes me crave more carbs and sugar and I just don't want to go down that path again. I've been heavy before. I don't ever want to go back there. I don't want to because getting six-pack abs means more to me. Not feeling sick all night means more to me.

You might not care about having six-pack abs. Maybe you just want to get off prescription medication, or you want your skin to clear up. Maybe you just want to play outside with your kids without feeling like you're gonna have a heart attack. You get to decide that those things mean more than a bowl of ice cream or half a pizza. You are worth more than that. You deserve more than that. Treat yourself like royalty. Feed your body and soul only the very best. Because you deserve it.

It all starts in the mind. You have to DECIDE YOU'RE WORTH IT. Then after a while, your body falls in line. It's a little like magic. When you stop eating carbs and sugar. When you stop putting chemicals into your body. You get used to it. Your body stops craving the junk and starts craving the good stuff.

I get it. Each year has a seemingly endless flow of food-based celebrations. Birthday parties, retirement parties, weddings. The list goes on. We've been trained since we were children to eat crap food at all of these occasions. I'm not telling you that you can't have those things. I'm offering you a choice. If you stick with me, eventually you will come to a point where you don't want them and it will be easy to just walk away.

The less you eat the crap, the less you'll want it.

In the short term, get into the habit of talking to yourself before you eat or drink anything. (You can do it silently, so people don't look at you funny.) When you get home after a long day of shopping and you just want to order a pizza, or when you're at that party and you're faced with sugary cocktails or cheese and crackers, say this:

I can have that _____ if I really want it. Right now, my body feels _____.

If I decide to eat/drink that, my body will feel _____.

Tomorrow morning, I will feel _____.

Do I really want it?

Then make a decision. Let me give you a hint. We all have different voices. Chances are, there's a big voice that says, "It's a special occasion. Go ahead—eat it!"

If you really pay attention, there's probably also a smaller voice. One that's quietly saying, "The last time you ate that, you were sick all night. Remember? Your stomach was cramping, and you felt like crap the next day. Maybe it's best to skip it." Or maybe it's saying, "But you promised this year would be different..."

Later in this book I'll give you strategies and tactics to "survive" those work conferences or parties and all the food, drink, and stress they bring, without gaining 10 pounds. The cool thing is that if you follow these strategies, chances are pretty good that you'll be able to attend all the special occasions you like, already adapted, and without the fear of gorging on cake. You'll be amazed how much easier it will be to say "I don't want it" every day after that.

## STRATEGY #2: BE YOUR OWN SUCCESS STORY

Have you ever watched a reality TV show? You know, the ones where people go into a private room and record "confessional" videos? They might be funny or they might make you cry, but those videos allow you into that person's real thoughts and feelings. The best ones are raw and full of emotion. The same can be said for success stories in weight-loss and fitness magazines, blogs, and TV shows.

The diet and fitness industries rely heavily on those emotional success stories to sell everything from pills and shakes to gym memberships and videos. We connect with success stories because chances are we're somewhere at the beginning. We can relate to the mom of three who used to be athletic but let herself get 40 pounds overweight. Or the bachelor who was always "the funny, fat friend" but could never get a date.

And what do we do when we read those stories? We feel like if they can lose the weight, so can we! We are in the same boat. If we just do the right things (or buy whatever that story is selling), then we'll be successful, too.

As powerful as those confessional videos and success stories are, nothing will ever be more empowering and inspirational than YOUR OWN SUCCESS STORY! That's right. Your before and after pictures. Your testimony about your own journey.

Here's the thing—only you know what will truly motivate you to finally lose the weight. ONLY YOU KNOW YOUR *WHY.* Maybe you just want to play with your kids without getting out of breath. Maybe you want to be intimate with your spouse and not wonder whether they're thinking about how fat you are. Maybe everyone in your family dies young from a particular illness and you don't want to be next. Deep down, you know why you want to do this. So let's tap into that well of inspiration and create a tool that will help you reach your goal faster than you can imagine.

I want you to create your own confessional video diary. Don't worry, no one is going to see it but you. All you have to do is go into a room (or maybe your car) and use your phone or a computer to record yourself. When you look into the camera, imagine you're talking to yourself. You are recording a message to the future you.

Now, Future You is definitely losing weight, but they might be sick and tired of this program. They're tired of measuring. They want to have a drink with the girls once in a while. They're ready to give in to temptation. They're about to go on vacation and completely blow all the progress you've made.

YOU are not going to let that happen.

YOU are going to give Future You a pep talk.

YOU are going to beg and plead for Future You to not give up. You're going to do whatever it takes to keep yourself on track!

I know this might sound silly, but hang with me here, okay?

The first video will probably be the most raw and emotional. I want you to explain to the camera exactly how you feel at that moment. Before you start the program—before you've lost any weight—describe how you feel.

How does your body feel when you wake up in the morning? Does anything hurt?

Do you feel drained all day long?

What about climbing stairs or picking up your children? How does that feel? What activities are you missing out on because of your weight?

What activities have you always wanted to try, but haven't because of your weight?

How do you dress? Why?

How do you feel on the inside? Are you hurting? Are you ashamed? Are you scared?

Is there someone you want to be proud of you? (Like say, *yourself*?)

Lay it all out. It's so important for you to draw a line in the sand and say NO MORE! You are never going back to your old way of life. You are becoming a new person and you need to vividly remember where you started from.

Your brain will play all kinds of tricks on you. It will try to sabotage your efforts. When you think back, your brain will make the details a little fuzzy. It will try to convince you that your heaviest weight wasn't so bad.

This video is your line in the sand. It's what you're going to come back to every time you think *it wasn't so bad*. I want you to lay out your pain in great detail. It's not fun, I know. You're probably going to resist it. Trust me. In a few weeks or months, you'll be glad you did it.

After you describe how you're feeling at the beginning of this journey, I want you to start talking about your hopes and dreams. Tell Future You what you're looking forward to. What activities will you take up? What kinds of clothes will you wear when you're smaller? How will your life be different? Paint this picture in glorious bold colors! Visualize exactly how you will look and feel when you lose this weight, and speak it aloud on the video. Help Future You remember the dream when they are about to cave in.

Finally, I want you to give Future You a pep talk. Beg and plead if you have to. Tell them not to give up! Tell them it's not worth cheating, not even once. Tell them you are counting on them to stick with the plan. Tell them you believe in them, and you believe in you, and you know you can do this. Say whatever you have to, and *say it with love.*

That's the first episode of your video diary. It might be short or it might be long. All that matters is that you are completely honest with yourself. All that matters is that you speak from your heart and give voice to the hopes and dreams you've been hiding inside. You know, the hopes and dreams you've been stuffing down deep with food. Let them come to the surface. The words are powerful. Speak them.

## THE REST OF YOUR VIDEO DIARY

You've just created an amazing tool. Anytime you feel like caving into temptation or you just want to give up, watch that video! Anytime you feel like your body has turned against you, watch the video. Anytime you just need a reminder of how far you've come, watch the video. Don't just record it and forget about it. Use it to motivate you and spur you on.

Future entries are up to you, but I encourage you to talk to Future You at least once or twice a month. Did you survive vacation without cheating? Awesome! Record an entry and talk about how proud you are of yourself. Did you zip up a smaller pair of jeans? Make a video! Record your celebrations and your setbacks. Record your ups and your downs. It's all part of the journey, and it will all help keep you going when you're having a challenging week.

There's one very important rule with your video diary—NO NEGATIVE SELF-TALK. It's not allowed! In your first "baseline" video, it's okay to describe how you're feeling, and a lot of it will probably be negative. After that, you must treat your body and your mind with kindness and respect. Your body has one job—to keep you alive, and it has done that job perfectly! Talk lovingly about yourself. Even if you're frustrated, use kind words. They are powerful.

In fact, I recommend you finish every video by looking into the camera and saying, "I love you" and "Thank you for taking such good care of me." It sounds kind of hippity-dippity, but it's not. Even if you feel ridiculous, do it anyway.

The more you get used to talking nicely to yourself, the more your body will respond the way you want it to.

## STRATEGY #3: PRACTICE MINDFULNESS

Most people get used to mindlessly shoving food into their mouths. We lick the spoon, we pick at our kid's plates, we open the bag of cookies and dig in.

I remember a day where I was super stressed out and to cope, I grabbed a big bin of almonds from Costco and just started mindlessly shoving them into my mouth. I'd eaten almost half of them before my husband walked by and saw what was going on.

"What are you doing?" he asked me, lifting the bin away. (I'm so grateful he's always got my back.)

I was stunned to see how many almonds I'd packed away without even realizing it. Mindless eating is something most of us have experience with, but it's simple enough to stop, and you do that by being mindful.

You'll notice I said it's simple, not that it's easy. You absolutely can do it. Be patient with yourself if you accidentally slip back into it, reset, and start again. It takes a hot minute to change something, even when you're aware of it.

See, we all go through what you may know as the scale of change. The first step on that scale is called unconscious competence. It means you don't know what you don't know.

Before you picked up this book, you were at step one. You didn't know the diet mentality had such a hold on you. You didn't know that your identity as "someone with a weight problem" has to shift to something else in order for you to get off the weight loss mountain once and for all.

As you started reading this book, you'll transition from unconscious competence to what's known as conscious competence. It's where you know there's a problem, but you don't yet know what to do about it. By *know* I mean you're starting to see why weight loss is such a struggle. You're starting to recognize ways in which you've sabotaged yourself. You're beginning to understand why unhealthy food seems to have such a hold on you. But you aren't yet sure what to do about it. By the end of this book, you will be sure what to do. When that happens, you'll enter step three: Conscious competence.

Conscious competence is when you know what needs to happen, and you know what you need to do about it, but it's not yet second nature. You have to think about it and work at it a little. You're creating your new normal, but it's not your normal yet. Conscious competence is where you've probably quit in the past. It is definitely the most challenging step for most people. You're forming new habits, you're making different choices.

In other words, you're being MINDFUL.

Stick with it, because without step three, conscious competence, you won't make it to step four: Unconscious competence. Unconscious competence means you no longer have to think about what you're doing. It's not work anymore, because it's second nature. It's your new normal.

It's also the step where you realize all the time and effort you put into reaching it was worth it.

Mindfulness is the key. Mindfulness is how you make it to step four, which, in this case, is living a happy, healthy life where you're no longer circling the weight-loss mountain.

## STRATEGY #4: DEAL WITH THE VOICES IN YOUR HEAD

The voices in your head are real! They mean well. They want to keep us safe and alive. You've probably got a cheerleader voice that says, "You got this. Keep going." Unfortunately, the negative voices that keep us stuck are usually the loudest. "What's wrong with me? Why can't I do this? I'm so weak!"

Sound familiar?

How about, "Just one bite won't hurt. You've already cheated once, you may as well keep going?" Does that one ring a bell, too?

Here's how to solve the "voices" problem: Don't try to defeat them. Instead, get them all talking to each other. Get them on the same page, working toward the same goal! Imagine the voices as real people and give them each a voice. Hold a "board meeting" and let them say whatever they want. Literally sit in a chair, become one of the voices, and talk. Then move to another chair, be the next voice, and let that one have its say. Move back and forth between chairs as long as you need to. Have a real conversation with yourself.

Remember, you are the one in charge. The negative voice may be loud, but YOU are the one in control. The cheerleader's voice may be quiet,

CRISTY "CODE RED" NICKEL | 79

but you can choose to ask them to repeat themselves over and over again, louder and louder.

If it feels weird to have a conversation out loud, you can write it out instead. Use different colors for the different voices. The point is to realize that you are having this conversation unconsciously all the time. These voices are ruling your life...but it doesn't have to be that way. You get to decide when enough is enough.

You can't just lock the voices in a closet or stuff them down deep inside you—they know when you're weak, and they'll always come back. So instead, let them talk, thank them for their viewpoints, and then you decide which voice to listen to.

Willpower isn't enough. You have to make a decision.

This is the last time you're going around this mountain!

## STRATEGY #5: KEEP A JOURNAL

Writing out your feelings on paper is a great way to get them out of you. It's also a proven way to shift into and solidify your new identity as someone who lives a happy, healthy life. Countless studies show that writing things out by hand leaves a neural impression that we do not get from typing or talking, which is why writing out affirmations, goals, and other positive outcomes and mindsets is so incredibly powerful.

Everyone's journal is unique to them. I've recorded details like when I finished my daily water intake, how I felt that day, things I did that I was proud of. That last part is important. Don't use your journal as a place to beat yourself up. It's a tool to help you manage your feelings, get them out of you, and write down the mindsets and actions that will help you get where you want to be.

It's okay to be honest with your feelings, but I want you to be supportive of and kind to yourself. No chewing yourself out in your journal (or at all), okay?

## STRATEGY #6: IMMERSE YOURSELF

Right now, you are immersed in habits, mindsets, and environments that are all contributing to your old identity. You are surrounded by people who want to eat all the time, even when they're not hungry. You're surrounded by snacks in the break room. You're surrounded by candy when you set foot in the supermarket.

The way to unravel all this unhelpful immersion is to start immersing yourself in something different. Immerse yourself in whatever will give your brain and body what they need to shift to your new identity. I've provided a wide variety of ways you can immerse yourself in the Code Red Lifestyle and stay connected to people who will lift you up. Reading this book is one way, but that's only the beginning. You can also check out my podcasts and YouTube videos, and read my blog posts. Download my app and take the Code Red Lifestyle with you wherever you go.

A committed accountability partner is another great way to help you immerse yourself in new information that will offset that old environment. Surrounding yourself with like-minded people is incredibly powerful. Get a group of friends or coworkers together and be Rebels together. You may need to make a few changes in your environment to help as well, such as clean out the junk food and replace it with delicious Code Red-approved foods, or stop buying soda and get yourself a really nice bottle for your water.

Once you start immersing yourself in this lifestyle, it's important you stick with it. Give it the opportunity to become your new normal, because right now, the pull of your old identity is strong. If you stop immersing yourself, your old identity will drag you right back to where you don't want to be.

Don't let that happen. Immersion will teach your brain a new way forward that does not involve having a weight problem.

## STRATEGY #7: MEDITATE AND OBSERVE YOUR MIND

Remember how I talked about listening to your body? Meditation is how you listen to your mind, and it doesn't mean you have to light candles and sit with your legs crossed for an hour. You can do that if you want, but all you really need is a few minutes.

Ideally, you'll settle in someplace quiet, without distractions, close your eyes, and breathe slowly and deeply. That's it. While you're meditating, let your mind wander where it wants to. The point is not to force your mind to be quiet. The point is to find a few minutes of stillness, so you can get in touch with your thoughts, kind of like a mechanic doing a check-up on your engine.

Noticing the thoughts that come up will show you which thoughts need your attention, such as where you might be sabotaging yourself. If no particular thoughts come up, that's okay too. Like I said, this isn't about forcing your mind to do something. If no particular thoughts come up, enjoy the stillness. It's very reenergizing. Even a couple minutes can make a huge difference.

Do what you can.

## STRATEGY #8: REWARD YOURSELF ALONG THE WAY

Let's talk about the power of rewards.

So many people tend to diminish their accomplishments. When it comes to celebrating how far they've come, they kick the can down the road and say, "I'll celebrate when..."

But "when" never comes, and before too long, they get frustrated and quit. The day-to-day process is where the magic unfolds. It's facing and overcoming the trials and tribulations that make it so rewarding to get to your next step.

Watching the dial on the scale tick down as you heal your life with real, nutritious food is one reward. That should make you feel awesome because it is a visible way to watch your progress in real time. Stepping on that scale is just as much a validation of your hard work as it is the first line of defense for keeping you on the right track. However, as wonderful as the weight loss is, it's important to remember that it's not all there is.

Rewarding yourself during the process is not only a powerful motivator, it keeps things fresh and exciting. It's an act of self-love. You are showing yourself that you are proud of you. You are proud of healing your body and healing your mind. You are proud of all the countless invisible benefits you are achieving by feeding yourself the right food. You are changing your thinking, and you are taking back your life.

As your body heals, you will eventually be able to trust its cravings, because it will be craving what it needs. Your body will perform better, your skin will glow. Now that's a reward! Your body is saying a great big *Thank*

*You.*That is the beauty of nutrition; it starts working right away. The sooner you feed your body healthy and wholesome food, the sooner you will begin to feel the rewards, but you can and should give yourself other rewards as well.

So how will you reward yourself for all your hard work? My first business coach clued me into this concept. I worked so hard to build up my business, and my coach had me write out every year what I was going to do to reward myself for reaching my goals. I planned shopping excursions. I planned trips with friends or family.

If you are used to thinking negatively about giving to yourself, you might be tempted to skip this. Don't! You are working so hard, and treating your body so well, you need to recognize that. The ultimate goal is always your health, but it is important to value your efforts as well. If someone in your life achieved a remarkable goal, you would reward them, so why not yourself?

You want to plan rewards ahead of time, and sometimes that can be difficult because we all have busy lives, but your hard work is worth it. Set multiple, achievable goals and a reward to go with each one. Lost 5 pounds? Go get a nice pedicure. Reached the 20 pound mark? Take a trip to the mountains with your sweetie (or all by yourself!). Since everyone has a different total number of pounds to lose, everyone's goals and rewards will be different.

Obviously, you want to reward yourself with something other than food. Part of the wholesome change you have made in your life is to no longer punish or reward yourself with food. So what are your interests? What makes you feel good? It could be going out and making some new additions to your wardrobe, or it could be a weekend at the spa. Maybe it's a pair of really nice noise-canceling headphones.

Set some time aside to figure out what will be the most rewarding to you, whether it's a weekend to go see a friend who lives far away, a new bicycle, dance lessons—whatever will help you feel good about your accomplishment. Whatever it is, you want that reward to look forward to as well as your ultimate goal.

Your body is healing and your health is improving, but when the scale isn't moving, people get frustrated. When that happens, look to your reward. It's a tangible thing to keep striving toward. I want you to keep working hard, I want you to feel encouraged and happy. When you do reach your next goal (like I said, reward yourself along the way, not just at goal weight), I want you to reward yourself because, guess what? You've earned it.

## STRATEGY #9: TRY NEW THINGS

One thing I see in people who reach their goal weight is that they really don't know themselves. Having a weight problem was such a huge part of their identity, that they have no clue who they are without the weight. You know what's awesome about building a new identity? YOU get to choose what that looks like! You get to decide what kind of clothes the new you wears. You get to decide what kinds of activities the new you likes to participate in.

Is the new you an outdoorsy type? Maybe start looking at camping and hiking videos.

Is the new you a dancer? Check out the local clubs or sign up for classes.

Does the new you want a garden, so you always have fresh food available to experiment with?

Maybe the new you takes a trip someplace new every month.

Trying new things along your journey can really help you. It's especially powerful if you choose activities that your old identity would have said "No way!" to, whether that's signing up for a new sport you've always wanted to try or wearing a sexy shirt you wouldn't have been caught dead in before.

Take a few minutes to write down a list of things you've always wanted to do, but that your old identity wouldn't let you. It can literally be anything. A ski trip to the Swiss Alps, wearing a bikini for the first time, or wearing a striking new shade of lipstick. Who is the new you? Start designing your new life now and ease into it as you go along. That way, you won't reach your goal and sabotage all your hard work just because you don't recognize yourself. Instead of looking in the mirror and thinking *Who's that?!*

You'll be saying, *Well hello there, gorgeous!*

What comes next is whatever you want. You get to create it for yourself, and that's freaking awesome. Choose some things you've always wanted to try, and make a plan to ensure they happen. Not only will it bring you so much joy, it'll help you discover (or re-discover) who you are without the weight.

## STRATEGY #10: FIND YOUR SUPPORTERS

Having community is HUGE in all areas of our lives, especially when we're going after a big goal like lasting weight loss. When you feel isolated and alone, you're a lot more likely to give in to old habits and mindsets that aren't serving you. You're a lot more likely to hear that old identity calling your name. A community where you can feel connected and supported by people walking the same path helps you stay committed to your new identity.

It breaks my heart when people disconnect from the Code Red community, because it's almost always a sign the pull of their old identity is overpowering their new one. Most of the time they don't even know it. Yes, there are a few outliers who can go it alone and do fine, but most people I see aren't like that. Most people need support outside themselves to do things like counteract the negative self-talk, pick them up if they fall, and share ideas and stories.

Another reason community is so important is because it provides accountability. There are very few people in the world who succeed at anything without accountability. When I say accountability, I'm not talking about paying lip service to reaching your goals. I'm not talking about people who will say nothing, or pat you on the head and let you get away with messing up over and over again.

I'm talking about people who say, "Look, I love you and I care about you, but I'm not interested in your excuses. I'm interested in what you're gonna do moving forward. What's your plan to do that?"

*That's* accountability.

Community also protects you from naysayers. You will have people in your life who support your decision to take your life back. But at some point, you may encounter people who do not. These are the people who nitpick what you're doing and try to convince you it's "unhealthy." They're the people who insist you have "just one bite," and take offense if you refuse. They're the people who passive-aggressively leave tempting junk food around for you to find, or put a slice of cake on your desk even though you already told them you're not interested. People may even say you look "horrible," or "too skinny."

Some naysayers may come around to your way of thinking in the long run. You may be surprised at how they start out critical, then watch your transformation for a while and come back wanting to know how you're doing it.

Either way, it's important to remember that no matter what they say, their antics are *not about you*. Seeing you commit to a healthy decision, like taking your life back, is a threat to some people. It may remind them they're not living up to their potential and rather than face that, they try to tear you back down to their level. It could be that eating is all you have in common with them and once you're saying "I'll pass" to Margarita Mondays with the girls, there's really nothing left for you to bond over. Some people are scared of getting left behind. The bottom line is that most people don't like change because it could be a threat and the fact that you are making a change is alarming to them.

Another thing to remember is that most people in your life have been putting up with your "dieting" for years, and even though they love you and want what's best for you, they're not ready to believe you when you say this really is the last time. That's okay. You don't need them to believe you yet. Stick with it and let your actions do the talking.

Do not let the naysayers derail you. Staying obese and sick because it's more comfortable for someone else makes zero sense and it's selfish of them to expect that of you. You can be compassionate about their discomfort, but you don't owe anyone an explanation about why you are taking YOUR life back.

Your community will have your back, even if some of the people in your life don't (yet).

Your community will celebrate you for saying no thanks to the cake, instead of taking it personally or looking at you like you spontaneously grew a second head.

Stay connected to the Code Red community. Let us lift you up and support you as you shift into this amazing new identity.

## IT'S TIME TO START YOUR SHIFT

Shifting away from seeing yourself as "someone with a weight problem" to someone who lives a healthy, full lifestyle is completely doable. Just know it's not going to happen overnight. After all, you've had this identity for a long time. But it absolutely can and will happen if you make the strategies and mindsets in this chapter a regular part of your life.

Here's a recap of the strategies you learned about in this chapter.

Strategy #1: Use Your Words

Strategy #2: Be Your Own Success Story

Strategy #3: Practice Mindfulness

Strategy #4: Deal with The Voices in Your Head

Strategy #5: Keep a Journal

Strategy #6: Immerse Yourself

Strategy #7: Meditate and Observe Your Mind

Strategy #8: Reward Yourself Along the Way

Strategy #9: Try New Things

Strategy #10: Find Your Supporters

Don't wait until you've lost all your weight to begin. You've got to start shifting into your new identity now, because the sooner you begin this shift, the more successful you will be, both in losing your weight and keeping it off...for good.

Holly Bergen
Millsborough, Oregon
Age 55
Lost 58 pounds

In 1965 when I was born, nobody was expecting spina bifida. People knew very little about the condition back then. It's a hole in your spinal cord. Because you artificially close the hole, your brain doesn't receive a signal to stop producing cerebrospinal fluid. They used to refer to us as "water-head babies," because our skulls would swell up from the excess fluid. Infant skulls are soft, so they expand until doctors put a shunt in to relieve the pressure.

Every case is different. Some people with spina bifida live their whole lives in wheelchairs. I spent the first 30 years of my life walking on crutches and braces. There were only three neurosurgeons in the entire country who knew how to do the surgeries to save my life.

When I was first born, some doctors said, "We can make her comfortable, but the best thing for her is probably if you just let her go to sleep and not wake up." Fortunately, our neurosurgeon did what it took to save me, which was to sew up my spine and put a shunt in.

I'm partially paralyzed from the waist down and completely paralyzed from the knees down. I have limited sensation between my waist and my knees, and no sensation from my knees to the tips of my toes.

My father built parallel bars in our basement—that's how I learned how to walk using something called a swing gate. He'd station my brothers on either end of the bars with M&M's or raisins to urge me forward.

God's wisdom is boundless and He put me with the best parents. Thanks to them, I did things no doctor would have imagined possible.

My dad told me, "Don't ever let anybody tell you you can't do something. If you wanna try something, you try it! Only you get to decide what you can't do."

A retired four-time Olympic swimming coach, my dad was inducted into the International Swim Coaches Hall of Fame. He didn't accept the words "no" or "can't". It also meant that my family's method for weight management was rigorous exercise and restrictive dieting. We didn't know any other way.

I was active. A swing gate requires that I bench press my weight every time I take a step, so while I carried extra body weight, I was fit. I climbed trees with my leg braces on. I would come back with skinned knees, arms, and elbows. My mom would ask why I didn't tell her when I was going to go do something like that. I'd reply, "Because you'd stop me."

I wasn't supposed to be able to tie my own shoelaces, feed myself, or even speak full sentences. I now have a BA in English and a MS in Counseling.

When I was 30, I developed an ulcer on my heel. The doctor I saw misdiagnosed it as a bone infection and blamed me for letting it get so bad. She never took an x-ray. She told my mother—in front of me—that I couldn't take care of myself or live on my own and to plan for me to be in a facility when they passed. She restricted me to a wheelchair for a year and a half, all the while mistreating the problem. During that time, I gained 50 pounds.

When you have a physical disability, you deal with grief and depression. To go from being as active as I was on braces to a wheelchair was crushing. I lost every bit of control over my body that a person could have.

Two years after the misdiagnosis, I saw an orthopedic surgeon who told me it was just a bone spur and I could've been back in my braces within two months. "Why didn't the original doctor ever take an x-ray?," he asked. I still don't have that answer.

By then I had gained so much weight, I couldn't get back on my braces without ruining my shoulders. I spent the next 24 years in a wheelchair, and developed a multitude of other health problems: hypertension, abdominal hernias, chronic fatigue, joint pain, inflammation, and stage one uterine cancer.

**I was just lost. I felt like giving up. I couldn't exercise, I couldn't starve myself. What could I do? I was truly hopeless.**

In 2002, I started seeing a naturopath. I lost 15 pounds, but only because I was starving myself. I told myself I wasn't hungry, but I was. The exercise and starving myself wasn't enough to get me out of the chair.

Although I lost some weight, I hadn't changed my relationship with food. I hadn't gone through that break in my thought pattern.

The following January, I saw this lady with a bright-pink mohawk on TV talking about diets, nutrition, and weight loss without exercise. That caught my attention. I thought *No exercise? No way!*

I bought Cristy's book and when the next 10-Pound Takedown challenge started, in February 2018, I decided to try it.

- In the previous six months trying things my way, I lost 2.4 pounds.
- Between January 26 and January 31 when I turned in my starting weight, I implemented the gallon of water a day. I lost another 2.4 pounds before the challenge even started.
- I lost another 17 on the challenge.

Two thirds of the way through the challenge I purchased a personal program on my credit card. My parents hit the roof over the cost (I thought my father was going to have a coronary) until they saw my progress in action. They realized, like I did, that it was the best investment in myself I'd ever made.

By the time I announced that I hit my goal I was actually .4 pounds below goal weight.

In the beginning, I ate more calories than I should have even though they were Code Red foods. At night, I thought I was hungry, but only because I hadn't adjusted to the rhythm of the new lifestyle yet.

I tripped up at a barbecue. I was eating right; salad with ranch dressing, a hot dog and hamburger—no buns. But they served cake, and I thought I could risk it because I'd been so good.

Within 20 minutes, I had awful stomach pains which lasted almost three days. I got right back on the horse after that. I had to listen to my body.

I couldn't believe it. I was having scrambled eggs cooked in butter, cream cheese, and bacon. (Newsflash: Fat does not make you fat; carbs and sugar do.)

I lost 58 pounds in a wheelchair!

Early on, I was skeptical. Massive weight loss without diet shakes, pills, prepackaged food or exercise? I was like "Okay, lady." But after it worked, I couldn't stop gushing about Cristy and her program. I'm overwhelmed by how much better my life is right now.

During a visit to my oncologist. He started looking around like he lost something and said "I was looking for the other half a person you usually bring!" The weight loss made me a better candidate for a hysterectomy to get rid of my uterine cancer. I was ecstatic about that, but he wasn't finished.

He said I'd lost so much weight that I no longer needed the surgery! Estrogen, which feeds the cancer, is created by excess body fat. So by dropping the weight, I was starving the cancer. He literally told me I was "killing it!"

He asked how I had been so successful with losing weight. I gave him my copy of Cristy's book, and explained the basics—how it's not keto or paleo, that it was basically sleep, water, and real food. I suggested that he share Code Red with other patients who needed surgery but were too overweight to have it done safely, and he agreed to put it in their hospital library.

Some people diet because they want to fit into a certain size of clothing or to look a certain way. I did it because I was sick, tired, and in pain. I was terrified because something in my body had the potential to kill me, and I was too heavy for the surgery to correct it.

I changed to save my life.

After six months on the program, my doctor said, "Keep doing whatever you're doing."

When I reached my goal weight, I purchased a red and white polka dot pinup dress. I saw myself in a full-length mirror and thought, *Wow—I'm kind of a dish!* I never expected that. I just wanted to feel better, to not be in pain, tired, sick, and afraid.

For people with physical disabilities who think it can't work for you, it can. If you take control of what you put in your mouth and get your sleep and water in you will take back so much control over your life. Anyone can reap the benefits of this program.

Drink the water, eat the food, get the sleep. Do everything they tell you to do. If you have any challenges, get support from the group.

Cristy wants to help you. She doesn't want lifetime customers—she wants to help you get the weight off and give you the tools to get on with your life.

If I can do it, you can too!

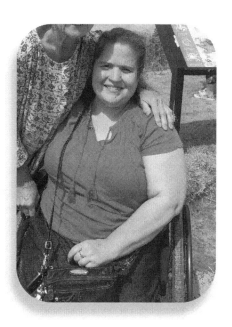

*Before*

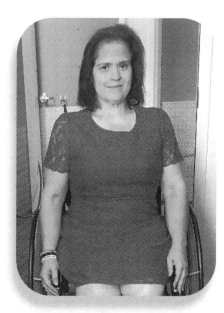

*After*

# CHAPTER 6

# THE CODE RED PROGRAM: HOW TO LOSE THE WEIGHT WITHOUT BEING HUNGRY

I T'S ONLY NATURAL to get all emotional about our bodies. After all, several billion-dollar industries are counting on us hating how we look. We've been brainwashed to believe there's something wrong with us ever since we could turn on the TV or pick up a magazine. Depending on how long you've been overweight, you may feel like your body is out to get you, like it's the enemy, like you're fighting a war. Often it feels like we're just outnumbered—our bodies are calling all the shots.

Why, oh why, do our bodies hate us?

Let's take a step back here for a moment and think. Your body is a complex organic mechanism. It completes thousands of processes just to get you through your day, and it takes energy to complete those processes, right? Your body is designed to store energy, just in case at some point there is no food to be found.

Let me say that again.

YOUR BODY IS DESIGNED TO STORE ENERGY.

It does that to keep you safe. To keep you alive when food becomes scarce. So you don't die! That energy is stored in the form of fat. Big deal, right? We all know that.

Well, consider this...

Maybe your body isn't the "enemy."

Maybe your body is perfect. It's doing its job day in and day out, regardless of how you feel about it.

You keep feeding it more calories than it needs for the day. It stores the extra in the form of fat, because someday you might need it. Only your body doesn't know that we live in an abundant society today. The majority of people have far more food than they will ever need. It's cheap and readily available any time of year.

We've become completely disconnected from our bodies. They go on about the work of converting the food we eat into the glucose (sugar) we need to survive, and storing whatever is left over. We go on about our daily lives, shoveling in more and more food out of habit or boredom or anxiety—but rarely because we're actually hungry.

What's really happening here is that we're storing up fat so we can survive during the next great famine. Except there isn't one. (Thank heaven!) So for years and years, we keep storing and storing. It's just a mechanical process. Yet we attach negative emotions to our bodies just for doing their jobs. It's hardly fair, but there is good news...

## YOUR BODY HAS A SECRET

Now what you may not realize is that your body is capable of running on two kinds of fuel—glucose and ketones. Sugar and carbohydrates break down into glucose, which is the easiest kind of fuel for our bodies to use. The process looks like this:

You eat a bagel. Your body breaks it down into glucose and uses some of it. Whatever is left over is stored as fat for later. This is an incredibly efficient process. Your body has been running on glucose most (if not all) of its life. It's very good at this conversion process, and it's very good at storing fat.

But what happens if you're suddenly shipwrecked and stranded on a desert island and have no access to starchy, sugary food? (Your cell phone drowned as you swam to shore, so there's no calling for help.) I call this the

Gilligan Scenario. You can fish. You can hunt. Eventually, the professor in you figures out how to open a coconut. But that's pretty much it.

Would you die? No. Not from starvation, anyway. Not for a long time. Because you have all this glorious fat that your body has been storing up. Finally—it's time! Your body gets to do what it was designed to do—change its fuel source to ketones and use up some (or all) of the stored fat. Ketones are energy that's created from fat.

It's kind of like a hybrid car that can switch from electric energy to gasoline. You store gas in the tank for when you need it. The car runs on electricity until the battery runs dry, and then you just push a button and switch over to a different fuel source. Your body runs on glucose until there isn't any more available, then it switches over to ketones. It makes ketones by burning stored fat. The longer and more efficiently you burn ketones, the more stored fat gets used up. And the less you weigh!

Go back and read that last paragraph again. It will change your life.

Seriously, I'll wait.

Now imagine you're back on the island, and you managed to rescue a waterproof crate full of Twinkies. (I don't know where they came from. Just run with it, okay?) Naturally, you're going to want to ration them. So you allow yourself just one Twinkie a day. The rest of the time, you eat fish and coconut milk.

Doing this, you're running on a little bit of both fuels. As you can imagine, it's not very efficient. Your body's engine never completely switches over to burning fat, so you just sort of sputter along. You're able to function, but you feel tired all the time. Maybe you have headaches and get grouchy.

This is what happens when you eat a so-called "healthy diet" by modern Western standards. When you consume foods that turn into glucose and foods that your body converts to ketones, your body is running on both kinds of fuel. Just not very well. It's also what happens when you switch back and forth between different diets, or when you allow yourself the occasional cheat. It's miserable!

Imagine for a moment what would happen if you could create the Gilligan Scenario on purpose, but in your own home, with showers and flush toilets and all your everyday comforts. What would happen if you chose to let your body switch fuels and burn fat for a while? What if you stopped feeding it grains and carbs and sugar, and switched to mostly healthy fat, some protein, and veggies?

I'll tell you what happens. Your body gets confused for a day or two. Is this for real? When is she going to go back to the bagels and doughnuts? Or should we think about switching over to fat? Hmm…not sure. Let's dump a bunch of water and see what happens. (The water flushes out and you lose several pounds right away.)

Then your body figures out that you're serious. The fuel source you're giving your body is high-fat and low-carbohydrate—perfect for creating ketones. Your body says, "Okie-doke! Time to switch over to fat-burning." And when you don't eat quite as much food as you need to survive, guess what?

## IT BURNS THE STORED FAT!

It doesn't happen overnight. It can take a few days or a few weeks for your body to fully convert to fat-burning mode. But once it does, you'll notice your energy levels soar. That brain fog that's been holding you down for months or years suddenly lifts. Your weight drops. Continually. As long as you consistently feed your body what it needs to burn fat, it will! Whether you have 10 extra pounds of fat stored up or 250—your body will use that stored fat as fuel until you tell it to switch back to burning glucose.

The reason you've been unsuccessful losing weight in the past is simply because you haven't switched your fuel source long enough.

Your body is perfect. It's been doing its job all along.

Its only goal is to keep you alive as long as possible. So stop hating it, okay?

If switching fuel sources sounds simple, that's because it is. Stop eating bagels and doughnuts and caramel macchiatos. Start eating eggs, bacon and broccoli. Drink water and sleep. Let your body burn up the stored fat. Done.

Take a deep breath. It really is that simple. We've proven it over and over.

When someone invests in a custom program, they fill out an extensive questionnaire so I get to know them and their individual needs. Then I write up a personalized nutrition program. After that, each client is medically screened by a registered nurse. Unless you get a custom program, I don't know your personal background. I don't know what you're sensitive to. I don't know if dairy makes your tummy hurt, or if you're a vegetarian.

So I'm going to give you the basics of the Code Red program here, and then I'll show you how to modify the recommendations to suit your needs, your taste, and your life. Most importantly, I'll show you exactly what to do to keep that weight off for good.

The books you're probably used to reading give you detailed restrictive instructions—meals to eat, recipes you're "allowed" to use, phases, and math formulas. If you haven't figured it out by now, this book is different. This plan is sustainable for your entire life, not just while you're losing weight. All you have to do to lose all the weight you want—and keep it off for good—is follow seven simple rules.

Now when I say follow the rules, I mean FOLLOW THE DAMN RULES!

You are strong.

You are a Rebel.

You keep to the code and don't stray. There's never an excuse to go off the plan. We don't believe in cheat days. We don't take weekends off. We don't stray just because it's someone's birthday.

Look, it's always someone's birthday or Christmas or an anniversary or something. You're going to get stressed. Loved ones will get sick and even die. Jobs will suck. Life isn't going to stop just because you're trying to lose weight. The world isn't going to stop turning. So that means you have to figure out how to stick to the rules in spite of whatever is going on in your life. The second you let yourself slide on one meal, it's a quick ride to a full-on binge. Or worse, you just give up altogether.

No.

We don't do that. One cheat will set you back a week of progress. If you don't think you can do this without cheating, think again! YOU CAN DO THIS.

You will need support, and that's why we have a strong community of Rebels. Every one of them has looked temptation and birthday cake in the eye and won. Every one of them has had a tough day now and then, days when they needed to vent and hear someone tell them to stay strong.

You want cheat days and gimmicks and *slooow* weight loss? Find another program.

You want this time to be the LAST TIME you ever have to do this? Follow the Code Red Lifestyle.

I know there's a good chance you've tried other ways to lose weight and failed. There's a good chance that deep down you are really afraid you'll fail again. That's normal. Please listen to me, though. You're not just learning a new set of eating rules. You're transforming both your body and your mind. You're choosing a path and sticking with it. When you make that kind of commitment, with the support of like-minded people, and you have a solid plan, you cannot fail!

You. Cannot. Fail.

## WHAT SHOULD YOUR GOAL WEIGHT BE?

If you're like most people I talk to, identifying your ideal weight is a confusing and frustrating experience. Your doctor is telling you one thing. Your insurance company might be telling you something different. There are government charts and scientific theories about what an ideal weight is for someone of your height. The magazines and TV advertising show you photoshopped models who are impossibly thin. Who knows how much those chicks actually weigh or what their thighs actually look like? There's so much conflicting information out there, how are you supposed to know what the heck your goal should really be?

One thing I've noticed is when I ask my clients what weight they think they should be shooting for, it's almost always at least 20 or 30 pounds higher than what I know they can achieve. They will pick a weight they know they can reach because they did it 10 years ago when they counted points and went to Dancercise twice a day.

They'll pick something they think is realistic for them, but isn't necessarily their ideal weight. If someone is 5'4" and, based on their custom program questionnaire, I can tell they should be around 130, they'll decide, "Okay, 175 sounds good to me!" And I have to tell them no, they can do better than that.

In the beginning, it's hard to believe when I tell them they can get down to where they were in high school. Some people have been overweight for so long, they don't even remember being a healthy weight. I get that. It's okay. Just realize that you can set "for now" goals. If you're 250, set a "for now" goal of 225 or 199. Then you can set another goal and another— as many as you need to get down to a number you can naturally maintain without a lot of struggle.

You can't hit a goal if you don't know what it is. So before we go into the rules, I want to help you get really clear on what number you want to hit during the weight-loss phase of this lifestyle. I've discovered something over the course of coaching for years and writing thousands of weight-loss programs: Everyone is different! There's no magic formula for what your weight should be.

I have a friend who is within half an inch of my height. Her ideal weight is 135, and mine is 154. When you see us each at our ideal weights, we both look great. I could never get to (much less maintain) her ideal weight and be healthy. And at my ideal weight, she looks very overweight. That's what I mean when I say everyone's different and there's no magic formula. And you know what else? Your body intuitively knows where it wants to be. It knows your number, and it might just shock the heck out of you when you figure out what it is.

So rather than looking outside yourself for your goal weight, try looking inward. Close your eyes and think back to a time when you were happy and you felt alive, strong, and healthy. When was the last time you felt truly sexy? It might be when you got married. Or maybe you were happy with your weight when you graduated high school. Now, about how much did you weigh then?

It's critical that you don't judge yourself on whatever number you come up with! If you currently weigh over 200 pounds, and you know you weighed 125 in high school, your gut reaction might be "Who the heck do you think you are? You'll never get back to that weight. That's in the past. You can't possibly get down to your high school weight. Stop aiming so high!"

But here's the thing—it could be that 125 is totally realistic for you. If that number feels good and right, then that should be your goal. Don't listen to that voice in your head telling you it's impossible.

You must feel good about the number you choose, even if it seems like you'll never get there. If you KNOW IN YOUR HEART that you felt amazing at 125— go for it! As you lose weight over time, your body is going to settle in right where it wants to be. There will be a place where you no longer have to struggle. A natural weight you can easily maintain. I don't know what your ideal weight is...and neither do you, right now. But you need to have a goal to shoot for. So it might as well be a goal that you have happy associations with.

As I mentioned, most people I work with set their goal weights higher than I think they should. They really want to be 140, but they can't remember a time when they weighed that little. So they shoot for 165, and that's totally fine! If they can recall feeling happy, healthy, and sexy at 165, that's a perfect goal.

What often happens is they reach that goal and start living the Code Red Lifestyle in maintenance mode, but they keep losing weight! They don't understand it. They go lower and lower without even trying. It's because they've healed their bodies with real, nutritious food. They're sleeping enough and drinking enough water and their bodies know where they want to settle. Maybe it's 150. Maybe it's 140, a number they couldn't even say out loud when they started.

You might also choose an initial goal that's too low. You'll know if that's the case because it will be really hard to stay at that weight. Your body will naturally want to settle a little higher. That's fine, too. The number on the scale is just a tool. It does not define who you are or what you're worth. You need the numbers to measure your progress and the direction the scale is moving is what matters. Are you going up or down compared to yesterday? After a while, the actual numbers don't really matter at all.

Your body is wise. It knows where you should be. So for now, set a goal that makes you happy. Just realize that might not be where you end up.

## WHAT IS "REAL FOOD" ANYWAY?

Processed food is anything you eat that has gone through a mechanical process before it gets to you, or comes from a bag, a can, or a box. It's food that has to be preserved somehow to be shelf-stable for long periods of time. Often it contains artificial chemicals and sugar to help improve flavor and texture, and preserve it for a longer shelf life. (Oh, and it probably has a TV commercial.)

Real food, on the other hand, appears in your grocery store pretty much like nature made it. Vegetables look more or less the same when you buy them as they did when they were picked. A steak has been through the butchering process, but it's still considered real food if the only ingredient on the label is beef. Breaded chicken nuggets, on the other hand, are highly processed, chemical-filled concoctions that may or may not have any actual chicken in them.

Food manufacturers want to sell you "food products," and they want to keep selling you "food products." They hire scientists to make them look, taste, and smell like real food. They hire scientists to make them addictive, too. The food-like products they engineer have the addiction built in to keep you buying. They'll market low-fat ice cream as healthy, but they'll add twice as much sugar as regular ice cream just to keep you eating it.

Have you heard of MSG? It's short for monosodium glutamate, and it is in 80% of the processed "foods" available to the average shopper. Hop online and google "MSG-induced obesity." To study obesity in mice, scientists feed them MSG to make them obese. Why are Americans eating what scientists give to mice with the purpose of making them obese? Your body doesn't need that. It doesn't need energy drinks, soda, processed "food," juice, or alcohol.

What your body needs is real food!

Here again, you've got to get used to reading labels and looking for the added sugar and chemicals. Frozen broccoli is technically a processed food. It comes in a bag. It's been through the flash-freezing process. But the only ingredient on the label is broccoli so it's considered a real food. It was broccoli in the field, and it's still broccoli, just frozen.

What's cool about frozen veggies is they often have higher levels of vitamins and minerals than the fresh versions in the produce section. That's because as soon as plants are harvested, they begin to lose their nutrients. So if it takes a week to get that broccoli from the farm to your table, there may not be much vitamin content left. When it's frozen right after it's picked, the freezing process preserves the vitamins and minerals until you eat it.

When you give your body nutritious, real food, it's not going to tolerate the processed, sugary junk food as much anymore. My stomach hurts after those rare occasions when I eat processed food. You will eventually find that you just don't want that stuff anymore. Instead of telling yourself you *can't* have that food, you'll be telling yourself you *don't want it*, and that's a beautiful thing.

That is the difference between good nutrition and a diet. Telling yourself "I can't have that" leads to a diet mentality. Diets have failure built into them; that's why there are so many of them. They're products, not lifestyles. On the other hand, nutrition is just giving your body what it really wants.

You will find that the Code Red Lifestyle is completely doable. It's not rocket science. All you're doing is reading labels and eating real food. By staying away from the processed garbage that our society is addicted to, you are healing your body. We live in a society that is overfed but undernourished.

Okay, are you ready?

## HERE ARE THE RULES

1. Sleep at least 7–8 hours every night.
2. Drink at least one gallon of water per day.
3. Weigh yourself every morning.
4. Don't eat past 6:30 p.m.
5. Get and keep the junk out of your house.
6. Follow the Foods to Eat/Foods to Avoid list.

I don't know about you, but I hate rules when I don't know why I have to follow them. Rebels will rebel. It's in our nature. So I want to help you understand why these are the rules and why YOU MUST NOT BREAK THEM. If you're serious about taking your life back, these are non-negotiable during weight-loss mode. We'll talk about how to keep yourself on track in a little bit. But first, you've got to understand the why.

## RULE # 1: SLEEP AT LEAST 7–8 HOURS EVERY NIGHT.

Sleep is the most important rule in weight loss. Even if you're doing everything else right, "if you ain't sleeping, you ain't losing."

Clients will insist to me they're doing everything right, yet do not understand why their weight loss has slowed, then add, "Well my sleep is off."

Saying that is like saying this:

"Cristy, I don't understand why my car won't start! I just put fuel in the tank, the engine gets regular maintenance, the oil's fresh, the key's in the ignition. I just don't understand what's going on. I mean, I haven't turned the key to actually start the engine, but why won't my car start?"

See what I mean? You have to get your sleep, and here's why.

When you don't get enough sleep, your body senses that as stress. It can't tell the difference between stress because you're being chased by a saber-toothed tiger and stress from a long work commute. Stress is stress. The first thing your body does to protect itself is hang onto fat. Fat means survival to your body.

My dad is a licensed counselor and we go around and around on this topic all the time. His clients really struggle with sleep and so do mine, but he believes that some people can function just fine on 5 or 6 hours a night. My experience has been that if people get fewer than 7 hours, their weight loss stalls out.

I think the key word here is *function*. Can you function on less sleep? Sure you can. You've learned coping mechanisms and trained yourself to manage that way—maybe for years. Perhaps you've even convinced yourself that you're just one of those people who doesn't need very much sleep.

I know that when I get fewer than seven hours a night, I get cranky easier. My skin starts to get blotchy and cellulite starts to show up. I notice my stress levels going up and my weight might go up too. What's worse, I start to crave sugar.

A word of warning for all you night owls and last-minute deadline workers: Lack of sleep will increase sugar cravings! What happens when you don't get enough sleep? It goes something like this: Your body says, "Hey, listen. You're hitting a wall. It's not looking good. You need to get some sleep."

And you say, "Hey. I've got crap to do. We've got to keep going."

Your body isn't stupid. It knows exactly what's going to happen...but you are pretty stubborn, and you keep pushing.

So your body says, "Okay. If that's the way you really want it, that's fine. If you're not going to sleep, then we've got to get some quick fuel in here to keep you going. You need a pick-me-up." And that's when the sugar cravings kick in.

It's just chemistry. It's how we're made. We make demands on our bodies, and we have to have fuel to support those demands. When we burn the candle at both ends, that fuel often comes in the form of sugar. A quick hit on a caramel macchiato. Oh, and you want to throw in a cookie with that? Sure, why not? You're working hard, you deserve it!

You will get that sugar high. The energy will be there for a little while. Then you're going to crash, and your energy will be lower than ever. If you keep ignoring your body, you'll need more and more sugar to keep going. Your weight will creep up. Your body will start to cramp and hurt. All because your body is crying out, "Hey! Take care of me! You're treating me like crap."

I can go years without a sugar craving, but sure enough, when I push myself too far, they'll come back. It's all too easy to fall into the downward spiral of sugar highs and lows. It's not worth it.

Starting right now, I want you to pay attention to your body. What does it really need? When it says, "Hey! Caramel macchiato! You need a doughnut. You just need a pick-me-up," that's your cue to pay attention, because that's a craving talking. Cravings are signs that your body really needs something else. Maybe it needs sleep. Maybe it needs some water. Maybe it needs to spend an evening laughing with friends. What it *doesn't* need is a doughnut!

It's okay to talk back to your body. You do it all the time when you ignore its warning signs. So next time those cravings show up and you just know you're pushing yourself too hard, try saying this:

"Hey there, body. Thanks for clueing me in. You're right. I am pushing you really hard. I have one errand left to do, and then I'll go home and take a nap. Okay? Help me get through this next hour and I will reward you with that sleep you need."

Maybe, just maybe—if you speak nicely to your body and treat it with kindness—it won't even bother sending those cravings...because you don't need that doughnut. Not even just one.

I know there are a lot of extra demands on you; everybody has them, but trust me, don't run low on sleep. You're not doing yourself any favors.

You're setting yourself up to fight a battle with your body and you already know the craving battle is practically impossible to win.

Follow the rules and get at least 7 hours a night, even if that means you have to rearrange your life a little bit. Make sure your room is cool, dark, clean, and free of clutter. If you have kids or pets in the bed, it might be time to do something different. Create a nighttime routine for yourself. It sends a message to your body that it's time to go to sleep soon.

Make your sleep a priority. Your body will thank you!

## RULE # 2: DRINK A GALLON OF WATER EVERY DAY.

What if I told you the biggest secret to losing weight and keeping it off? What if I told you it wasn't exercise? It's not shakes and pills. It isn't a diet. What if I told you it was free? It is available to you right now, and you can start seeing results and feeling better immediately.

What if I told you that? Would you believe me?

I've been in this industry since 1994. I competed in three body-building competitions. While studying exercise physiology at the University of Memphis, I took up professional boxing as a way to pay for books and tuition. I was named one of the top three most dangerous females on the planet. I've written thousands of nutrition programs for people all over the world. So yeah. I know what I'm talking about when it comes to nutrition and losing weight, and I want you to hear the truth.

You ready for my non-secret?

WATER.

Let me say that again.

Water.

Drink a gallon of water every day.

It sounds simple, doesn't it? It sounds too good to be true, I know. It's not. There are so many positive correlations between water consumption and good health. Not only does it help your hair and nails grow, but it also helps you sleep. It helps regulate hormones. It gives you energy. It's going to keep you full and satiated for long periods of time.

Water consumption is absolutely key to weight loss and keeping your weight down. Try it. You won't want to have those caramel macchiatos. You won't want the candy, the cake, or the other unhealthy treats you normally crave.

Why haven't you heard how much just plain old water can help with your weight loss? Because there's no money in it. Water is free. (Thank goodness!)

Here's the deal—when you're thirsty, your body sends signals that it's hungry. So, very often you eat instead of drinking. But 9 times out of 10, you're not hungry. You are just dehydrated.

Here are some of the main benefits of drinking a gallon of water a day:

YOU FEEL FULL. And there won't be room in your tummy for the junk.

YOUR BODY FLUSHES OUT TOXINS. Your kidneys eliminate toxins and waste products from the blood and urine, and process water-soluble toxins from the liver. If you don't drink enough water, your kidneys won't have enough fluid to function properly.

YOU HAVE AMAZING ENERGY. The number one reason for daytime fatigue is dehydration. So staying hydrated may help you have more energy. Since your brain is mostly water, drinking plenty of it helps you concentrate and be more alert.

YOU SLEEP BETTER. Staying hydrated allows your brain to work at its best, even when "working" means "resting." A well-hydrated brain lets you enjoy a good night's sleep and wake feeling rejuvenated and ready for the day ahead.

YOUR SKIN CLEARS UP. Drinking water keeps your skin moisturized, fresh, soft, glowing, and smooth. (Psst! Good hydration also helps get rid of wrinkles.)

YOUR HAIR BECOMES HEALTHIER. If your hair follicles lack water, your hair will become dry and brittle. This gradually slows down and even stops the growth of your hair.

Now, a gallon of water is a lot to drink if you're not used to it, but it's completely safe. Can you drink too much water? Yes. It's called hyponatremia and it happens when your electrolyte balance gets out of whack.

The rule of thumb is that you need half your body weight in ounces of water just to maintain minimal body function like tear ducts, sweat glands, urination, saliva, etc. To aid in weight loss, you want to add to that because you're cutting out all the energy drinks, sweet tea, and even water-filled fruits that you normally consume. So you need to add the water to thrive.

A gallon of water is 128 ounces, which is a pretty safe amount for most people. If you're exerting yourself on a really hot day, your body may ask you to drink more water. Listen to your body.

Some people don't like the taste of water. I hear that from my clients all the time. There are a few good ways to get all those ounces down easier. One simple way is to use a straw. Straws make you drink faster. (Why do you think restaurants give you straws? So you'll finish the first drink quickly and order another one.)

Use the ten-sip method. Every time you pick up your water bottle, take ten sips through your straw. You'll be amazed by how much easier it is to get your water in.

Drink your water at room temperature. Ice-cold water is a lot harder for most people to get down.

Here are some things you can add to your water to give it a little flavor: Lemon slices or lemon juice, lime slices or lime juice.

You can also put a tea bag in your water. I'm talking about a normal tea bag, not powdered instant tea with added chemicals and sugar. Tea bags come in a massive variety of flavors, and will give you plenty of variety.

Another thing you can add to your water is an electrolyte supplement. There are two you can use: Ultima, or Re-Lyte, from Redmond Real Salt.

Just don't be tempted to turn your water into Kool-Aid, even with these electrolyte supplements. It's fine to add a scoop of Ultima or Re-Lyte, but don't get carried away.

Water. It's simple. It's free. It's available. It starts working immediately. Drink a gallon of water today and each day after that. I promise you will thank me for it.

## RULE # 3: WEIGH YOURSELF EVERY MORNING.

People have a love/hate relationship with the scale. No matter what number shows up, they either feel happy or they beat themselves up. Doing that is like looking at a thermometer and beating yourself up because of what the weather is outside.

Conventional wisdom says you should only weigh yourself once a week or even once a month. Code Red Rebels weigh themselves every single day. Even when they're traveling or on vacation. (We pack travel scales, in case you were wondering.)

Daily weigh-ins are part of the Code Red Lifestyle because the scale is your first line of defense. It's your first clue that you're either on track or you may need to tweak something you're doing. If you only weigh yourself once a week, and your weight goes up, how are you supposed to figure out what went wrong? If you binged on a bag full of Oreos earlier in the week, it's pretty obvious what happened, but what if you did everything right? It's really hard to figure out what's going on if you have to analyze seven days worth of data.

If your weight goes up after just one day, it's pretty easy to see what's happening. Maybe you didn't get enough sleep, or you fell behind on your water. Maybe you ate something that didn't agree with you and your weight went up, or maybe you're just really stressed out at work.

I had one client whose weight suddenly went up for a few days in a row. She was logging everything, and getting all her sleep. It didn't make sense that she was gaining. We looked at her log carefully and noticed that she had just started adding flavoring to her water.

The sweet taste of that flavoring made her want it all the time. So instead of a tiny bit in her water now and then, she was using a lot of it in every bottle of water she drank. I had her cut that stuff out, just as an experiment, and sure enough her weight came right back down.

If she had waited to weigh in for a week or two, who knows if we would have figured it out so quickly? She might have continued to gain, lost confidence, and quit the program altogether.

Instead, we were able to troubleshoot the problem in just a day or two. She recognized exactly why she was gaining. Something weird was happening and we just had to figure it out. There was no stress, and no blaming herself for being "bad" or "screwing up." We just worked on the problem. Pretty refreshing, don't you think?

The only thing that matters is the *direction* the scale is moving. Let's say you made a mistake and mindlessly licked the spoon while making cupcakes for your kid's birthday party. If you see a gain first thing in the morning the next day, guess what? You're going to buckle down and make sure you follow the rules. You're going to course correct immediately. If you wait for a week, who knows how much damage you'll do before you get back in control. Daily weighing means daily accountability. It's not about the number itself, it's about that *overall trend*. We want it to be trending down.

Daily weighing also means that you will eventually make peace with your scale. Remember, this is a new way of life, not a diet. Which means you're going to be weighing yourself every day for the rest of your life, ideally. Even when you're at goal weight, the scale is still your first line of defense. So rather than hating the scale, or getting mad at it, after a while it's just going to be a thing you do first thing in the morning. No big deal. The numbers will eventually cease to grab hold of you and affect your whole day. It might take a while, but at some point, your scale will become a companion—not a source of shame or guilt, and not something to obsess over.

Here's how I want you to weigh yourself.

First, get yourself a good digital scale, one that weighs down to the ounce. If your bathroom scale is 10 years old, do yourself a favor and get a new one. You deserve it. This little guy is going to be with you for an amazing journey. You do not need a fancy one that claims to measure body fat percentage, heart rate, and other facets of your health. Not only are those scales highly inaccurate, they distract you with additional information you don't need.

Every morning when you wake up, go potty to get rid of the water you drank yesterday. Then strip down naked and weigh in. Do this before you eat or drink anything! And when I say naked, I mean it. My mom even takes her Fitbit off because she swears that thing weighs a pound. Then, as soon as you weigh in, log your weight. Code Red's custom program clients are required to log theirs in the Lose-It app, but you can keep a little notebook by your bed, or print out the weight-tracking sheet you get in the Code Red Starter Kit mentioned in the beginning of this book. It's up to you. The important thing is to do it every single day.

What happens if you're up from the day before? We'll talk about that in a little bit. There are very specific reasons for weight gain. And once you know how to troubleshoot what's happening, you'll know exactly what to do to fix the problem without blame, shame, or guilt. For now, though, let's keep going through the rules.

## RULE # 4: DON'T EAT AFTER 6:30 P.M.

This one rule gets the most pushback. Why 6:30? Is it like Cinderella? Will you magically turn back into a pumpkin if you eat past 6:30?

The technical answer is that you want to go to bed a little bit hungry. You want your body to be done with the major digestive functions by the time you go to sleep, so it can focus on all the other processes it has to do at night, like deep healing and hormone regulation.

Some people say, "Can't I just make sure I eat 3 hours before I go to bed?" and you would think that's a reasonable solution, but my years of experience say no. If it were up to me, I'd have everyone finish eating even earlier, like 5 p.m. I usually finish my last meal at 4:00. (But then, I'm usually in bed by 8:00.)

There's just something about 6:30. It's the latest time I can push and have people still lose weight the next day. I'll see custom program coaching clients ask why they didn't lose the night before, only to admit they ate at 7:00 or 8:00. Eating that late is the answer to why they didn't lose. Every time. Even if they went to bed later. I don't know why it is. It just is.

If you work the night shift, or you typically stay up past midnight, first make sure you're getting enough sleep. Then adjust that 6:30 number to be at least three hours before your normal bedtime. I would prefer you stop eating 4 or even 5 hours before.

Remember, the goal is steady weight loss. You can even see a drop on the scale every single day. Just follow the rules, and your weight will go down.

## RULE # 5 FOR HEAVEN'S SAKE, DON'T KEEP JUNK FOOD IN YOUR HOUSE!

Set yourself up to succeed. If there's ice cream or cookies (or for me, tortilla chips) anywhere in the house, you're going to cave in and eat them at some point. You might be able to resist once or twice, but sooner or later, that willpower is going to let you down.

Rebels live in a safe zone. That means cleaning out your cupboards, your refrigerator, your freezer, your "secret snack stash" in the car—everything! All the sugar. All the starchy carbs. All the alcohol. If we don't eat it on the program, get it out of your environment.

Now, I realize you may not live alone and your family may not be on board with your new lifestyle (yet). So what do you do if your spouse simply must have cold beer in the fridge? Or your kids can't live without their afternoon snacks? There are solutions.

The first thing you need to do is explain to them that you are serious about this new lifestyle and you need their help and support. You'll be amazed how helpful your family can be when you just ask. Then create some success strategies.

If your roommate needs that cold beer, consider getting him a mini-fridge and keeping it in the garage. If it's a huge temptation for you, have him put a padlock on the door. I'm totally serious! That's not weird. It's smart. Maybe your kids could eat their snacks at a friend's house, or you could stop for a treat on the way home from school. The whole idea is that your home is safe. There's no temptation there.

Do you always grab a doughnut and coffee when you stop to get gas? Have your spouse keep the tank full for you. Or pay the extra two cents to go to a full-service gas station so you don't have to get out of the car. There's always a way to avoid the temptations. Get creative!

Okay, so what about when it's a holiday or special occasion? Same deal. No junk in the house. If you're hosting a party and there's tempting food there, fine, but the leftovers either go home with the guests or in the trash. If well-meaning friends drop by with a container of cookies, you don't have to insult them by refusing the gift, but get it out of the house as soon as they leave. Give it away. Take it to work or just throw it away.

THIS IS YOUR LIFE. YOU ARE THE BOSS. If there's no junk in the house, you don't have to wrestle with your willpower. You'll be just fine.

## RULE # 6: FOLLOW THE FOODS TO EAT/FOODS TO AVOID LIST.

This is where your decision to take your life back really begins. There's no way around it. You will have to avoid certain foods during weight-loss mode.

Ideally, some of these things will never make it back into your diet, but for now they are definitely off-limits. Rather than listing 10 pages of individual foods, I'm going to group most of the foods into categories—like avoid grains, avoid alcohol, avoid cheese, etc.

The best way to succeed with this is to KEEP IT SIMPLE! Remember, you have to measure and weigh everything that goes into your mouth. You have to keep track of it all, and several major categories of food will be eliminated during weight loss mode.

The fewer ingredients in a meal, the better. It's much easier to weigh and log a hamburger patty with lettuce, tomato, and no bun than it is to figure out what's in an "approved" shepherd's pie. Complicated recipes with lots of ingredients are just difficult. Stick with meat, eggs, vegetables, nuts, seeds, seafood, and fat. Make it easy on yourself.

If there's a food you're considering eating, and you're not sure if it's on the approved list, ask yourself two questions:

How much sugar does it have?

Does it have enough fat to keep me full?

If it's low-sugar and has a good amount of fat (or you can add fat to it), then it's probably fine. If it's high in sugar or highly-processed, don't eat it!

I'm the kind of person who could just eat tuna out of a can every day for a month and be totally fine, but you're not me. If you need variety, keep a list of meals you love, and rotate them in often. If you log a meal in LoseIt once, it's stored forever. Use the tools available to you.

I've made a printable foods list available to you in the Free Code Red Starter Kit I mentioned at the beginning of this book. It lists categories of foods to eat and foods to avoid. Print it out and post it where you will refer to it often. For now, you can find the list on the following page.

| OKAY TO EAT | AVOID THESE |
|---|---|
| **Berries** (blueberries, blackberries, strawberries, raspberries, huckleberries) | **Grains** (including quinoa, rice, oatmeal, corn) |
| | **Any breading on food** |
| **Full Fat Dairy Items** (Greek Yogurt, Cottage Cheese, Cream Cheese, Sour Cream, Heavy Whipping Cream) | **Pasta** |
| | **Milk** (whole, skim, or otherwise) |
| **Any Vegetables** | **Processed/Prepackaged Food** |
| **Any Meat** | **Cheese** |
| **Unsweetened Nut and Seed Milk** (cashew, almond, hemp, flax) | **Sugar** |
| **Seafood** (not breaded) | **ANY Soda or ANY Juice** (diet or regular) |
| **Nuts & Seeds** | **Any Type of Potatoes** |
| **Eggs** | **Yams** |
| | **Sweet Potatoes** |
| | **Corn and Corn Products** |
| **Healthy Fats** (olive oil, coconut oil, avocado, butter) | **Fruit** (other than the berries listed) |
| **Mayonnaise** | **Lentils/Legumes** (including peas, peanuts/peanut butter) |
| | **Alcohol** |

Jade Gallagher
Fairfax, Vermont
Age 32
Lost 74 pounds in 5 months, maintained since September 2018

I was never super heavy growing up, but I always felt like the short, chubby girl. At 4' 11", I don't have anywhere to hide extra weight. Twelve years ago, I had the first of four kids, which started that "new mom" body that stored fat like a pro. Later, I was put on medication and my weight ballooned out of control.

I've had psoriasis for over 15 years, but psoriatic arthritis wasn't diagnosed until 2016 or so. It inflamed my joints causing scar tissue to build up. It spread so quickly, within two years it was all over my body. It got so bad I couldn't use my hands, hips, or knees without terrible pain.

Even the simplest things were impossible—things I love doing. I couldn't even hold a hairbrush to brush my daughter's hair. I couldn't tuck my kids in at night, because I couldn't get upstairs. I couldn't cook dinner, because I couldn't hold a spatula or flip a pancake. My hands just wouldn't work.

I'd exhausted every medical option available in the US to manage psoriatic arthritis pain—countless steroids, day-long infusions at the hospital every couple of weeks, even chemotherapy drugs. I gained a lot of weight taking those medications, especially the steroids.

I asked my doctor how to lose weight, sure that a medical professional could help. She looked me over and said, "Well, you need to exercise more and eat less."

I couldn't even walk upstairs! How was I supposed to exercise? I felt completely defeated.

To lose weight, I tried shakes, diet pills—anything I could get my hands on. If it promised weight loss, I tried it. I even resorted to seeing a doctor in the hope of receiving injectable weight-loss medicine.

I drove six hours to see the nearest weight-loss doctor to find that he required his patients to consume protein bars and shakes for six months before the injections. I had to pay $6,000 before I could even be considered for the injections.

I left his office with a bag full of those protein shakes and bars, embarrassed and deflated. To soothe myself, I went straight to a gas station and bought a massive chocolate chip cookie and a Mountain Dew. When I tried the protein shakes, they were disgusting. I canceled my future appointments.

I was headed for a wheelchair because of my pain. My husband and I discussed how to make our house wheelchair-accessible. I had to give up our clothing business because I couldn't even put a shirt on a hanger. My husband is active-duty military, so there was no way he could run the business alone.

The latest set of labs from my doctor indicated that all the medications I was taking had put my liver into complete failure. I had to stop taking them all immediately. We'd exhausted all options for treating my condition.

Shortly after that, a friend of mine from Alaska posted pictures from her vacation on Facebook. I immediately noticed she'd lost weight. It had only been six months since I'd last seen a photo of her. I asked her which weight-loss drugs she was taking and which doctor she was seeing. I was ready to fly to Alaska to get access to her doctor.

She laughed and said she was just eating real food, sleeping, and drinking water. On top of losing weight, she said that it was healing her immune disorders too.

I was skeptical about the healing part. All I cared about was losing weight. That night, I ordered Cristy's book. Once I had it, I went shopping and stocked up on Code Red foods. The book suggested keeping a video journal, so on the way back from the grocery store, I recorded my first entry.

**For the first time in a long time, I felt hope.**

In my first two weeks following the book, I lost 10 pounds. I was blown away! It had taken nine months to lose three measly pounds gagging down those nasty shakes.

Two weeks later, I ordered a custom program. I knew I needed support and accountability. With all my medical issues, I wanted another person's hand in it to make sure everything was okay.

I had a moment of buyer's remorse, but then I thought about all the money I'd wasted on shakes. The results I'd gotten from those were nothing compared with two weeks following Code Red.

As a hard-core sugar addict, my detox period was brutal. I felt like I had the flu and I had a massive migraine that lasted almost nine days. Before Code Red, I treated migraines with over-the-counter medicine and Cola. This time, I knew drinking soda would reset the detox process. I stayed Code Red-compliant, and it paid off.

I woke up on Day 10 of my custom program and realized, *I'm not in pain anymore. Whoa!*

I had an infusion treatment scheduled for the following week. The treatments—which were destroying my liver—were for pain I didn't have anymore, so I called in to cancel. I told her I'd changed my eating habits and was pain-free. I said I'd call her if I needed another appointment.

A few months later, test results showed that my liver was healing. Considering I had been a candidate for a liver transplant, that was incredible news. I couldn't wait to share Code Red with my rheumatologist. Her response shocked me.

"I'm so proud that you're eating healthier. However, I would not say that your eating has anything to do with your psoriatic arthritis not being inflamed."

That was the only thing that had changed—how could it be anything else? Still, she insisted psoriatic arthritis was incurable, and only treatable with medication.

**It's baffling to me that the highest-ranked rheumatologist in New England didn't see the connection between my lifestyle change and the disappearance of my psoriatic arthritis pain.**

Later, blood work indicated that my liver was completely healed. My blood pressure is lower than it's ever been. I feel better now than I felt at 16, when I was an athlete and cheerleader.

When I began following Code Red, it was like a switch flipped in my brain. Before, I'd always grasped at any excuse to cheat, but none of that infiltrated my Code Red journey. I was completely no-nonsense and stuck to the rules. When I traveled, I took my meals with me. I planned and prepared.

My biggest struggle was sleep. I'd always been a light sleeper, but for the first few months of Code Red, I never felt like I was getting enough. I'd wake up at 5:00 a.m., even though I'm not an early morning person—my body was just ready to go. My coach suggested I go to bed earlier, and that worked.

My family was very supportive, especially my husband. He helped me clear out our pantries and fridge. We have four kids, and our youngest son struggled with attention disorder. I read that removing sugar from his diet could help. With Code Red, he is able to concentrate better. He has even moved beyond age-appropriate learning and is now doing multiplication and reading chapter books. If he eats sugar or grains, his attention suffers. Once those foods are out of his system, his focus improves.

**My husband and I agreed that becoming a Code Red family was the right choice.**

Our house is a Code Red safe zone. Our kids eat Code Red-approved foods for breakfast, lunch, and dinner. They take Code Red-approved lunches to school. I found ways to make the switch fun for them, like fixing pancakes with sugar-free chocolate chips. I give them options, but only between healthy foods.

My husband was overweight too, and I really struggled with that. I wanted him to feel the newfound energy I was enjoying. He ate Code Red at home, since that's all we had, but wasn't making an effort to lose weight. Later, I learned it was because he wanted to focus his energy supporting me. Once I reached my goal and entered maintenance, he decided to finally focus on himself. He lost over 50 pounds and weighs less now than he did coming out of bootcamp.

Code Red impacted my family in a huge way. My brother lost about 70 pounds just from reading the book, and my aunt lost about 80 pounds. Many of my extended family have lost significant amounts of weight following this program.

In maintenance, I reintroduced foods to see how they would affect me. I've identified which foods cause my psoriatic arthritis to flare up, so I avoid them. I rarely go off plan, because it's so easy to revert. I never want to be back there again.

The connection to other Rebels is huge because it keeps me in the right mindset. Otherwise, it would be really easy to go on a binge and gain a bunch of weight back. Knowing that this group will hold me accountable keeps me on track.

**One of my favorite things about this lifestyle has been rediscovering my love of shopping.** I used to be embarrassed about the clothing sizes I had to purchase.

I've rediscovered my love for myself, which allows me to love others in a way that feels more genuine. Before Code Red, it was difficult to express to anyone how much I truly loved them. I've discovered the self-confidence to step up, speak out, and love those around me in a deeper way.

If you are considering Code Red, consider WHY you want to lose weight, because that plays a huge role in your drive to succeed. Start by reading the book or trying a challenge. When you're ready, a custom program is the fastest way to get the weight off.

Code Red gave me my life back. More than that, it gave me a life I never dreamed of.

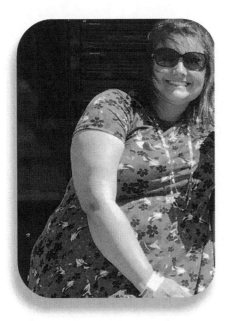
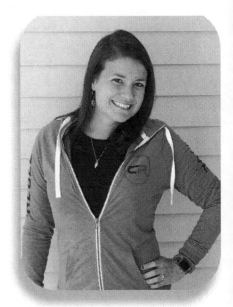

*Before*                         *After*

# CHAPTER 7

# WEIGHT-LOSS MODE

HERE WE GO! Weight-loss mode is a state of mind for Code Red Rebels. It's where you stick to your guns, no matter what. Christmas, birthdays, deaths in the family—none of these matter. You find other ways to celebrate and deal with stress. Weight-loss mode is where you get to stand in your power. You have the power and you have the control to handle this. Trust me, you do!

This isn't some quick-fix 30-day plan. You stay in weight-loss mode until you reach your goal weight. For some people, it might be 30 days. For others, it might be several months, but if you stay strong and rely on the Code Red community for support, it will take a lot less time than you might think. Every person is different, but I have Rebels who lose 1/2 to 1 pound a day with no trouble, and they are *healthy!*

Remember, you're in charge of how fast and how long your body is using fat for fuel. If you cheat once, you've switched your body back to burning glucose, and it can take up to a week to switch it back over. Stay strong.

## YOU'RE NOT GOING TO STARVE

Over the course of your weight-loss program, you will gradually consume fewer and fewer calories. You might be surprised by this, but in today's society, people need a lot fewer calories than they think.

I know that sounds like bad news. If you're used to eating 5,000 calories a day, the idea of dropping it down is scary. The good news, though, is you will lose weight. If your body is used to 3,000 calories, then it will naturally lose weight when you cut that number down and give it the right foods. As you lose weight, you are going to eat less, and that is okay, because your body changes as you lose weight.

In the first week, you're going to eat a lot of calories. Guaranteed. It's a natural reaction, because your body is getting used to a new way to eat and it's hungry. Often, in week two, people notice a natural decrease in appetite. I'll hear things like "Wow. You know, I had budgeted myself two eggs and four strips of bacon, but I only had one egg and three strips." That is a sign of someone naturally feeling less hungry. That's good. Forget the clean-plate club. Never force yourself to eat if you're not hungry.

My mom doesn't like to eat breakfast. She has just never been very hungry in the morning, so she doesn't eat until 11 a.m., and then she's good until about 5 p.m. Personally, I don't like to eat late. I'll eat meal one in the morning and meal two in the afternoon, but I find that I don't really need that evening meal. There is no cookie cutter method.

Everyone is going to eat their meals differently. The fact is, you will eat less as you adjust to this program. Don't force calories.

If you're into weeks 3 and 4, and the weight is not coming off, it typically means you're forcing yourself to eat more calories. It's okay not to eat the full amount all the time. The rule of thumb is this: If you're not hungry, don't eat.

Sometimes people ask me, "But Cristy, what about starvation mode? Won't I tank my metabolism if I eat fewer than 1,200 calories? Won't my body start holding onto fat if I don't eat 6 times a day?" They are genuinely scared that their bodies will shut down and not lose weight if they don't eat that magical 1,200 calories.

First of all, everyone has a different number of calories they need to survive based on their age, weight, activity level, and basal metabolic rate. That's the reason that I have to calculate precise numbers of calories and fat/carb/protein ratios for every custom program. There's no magic number that works for everyone.

The whole starvation mode idea, and the notion that you need to eat 6 times a day, these are more lies we've been told by the food industry. Think about it. Who benefits when we eat more food? Umm...the people selling us that food! The truth is you probably don't need that many calories. You need energy.

When you're eating high-fat, healthy foods like avocado, you get twice as much energy and nutrition per gram of food. Which means you don't need the same volume as when you were eating sugar and simple carbs. Your brain may want to eat more. Your eyeballs might miss the big plates overflowing with mashed potatoes and gravy. Your emotions might want dessert, but your physical body doesn't need it to survive.

If you're really low on calories, like 500 a day for 30 days straight, then yes, you could possibly damage your metabolism. But if you're truly listening to your body and feeding it real food, it's unlikely you'll get to that point. Your body knows what it needs. If you're overweight, then it needs to burn off all that extra energy you've been storing as fat. Listen to your body. Are you actually hungry? If so, eat a high-fat meal. If you're not, don't eat.

## WHAT YOU SHOULD EXPECT THE FIRST WEEK

The first week is gonna be hard. I'm not going to lie to you (ever). When you've been eating a standard Western diet full of sugars and grains and caffeine and chemicals, your body needs to detox all that crap out of your system. It ain't gonna be pretty. Don't let that scare you, because you are strong and you can get through it! I think it helps to know what to expect, but realize that it's different for every person. Not everyone experiences this stuff, and you might get through the first week without a problem.

Here's the thing—sugar is eight times more addictive than cocaine. So depending on how much sugar you've been consuming and how hooked you are on those sodas and snacks, you can expect your withdrawal symptoms to be similar to withdrawing from narcotics. You might experience headaches, nausea, shaking, achy joints, a foggy head, and/or extreme fatigue. You might be so exhausted you can't function at all.

Many people describe detoxing from sugar and grains as having flu-like symptoms. You're going to be hungry and grumpy. Little things might start to bother you. If you've been consuming 4 or 5 sugary sodas a day and you switch to plain water, of course you're going to feel like crap for a little while. The symptoms can last just a few days or up to a week or more.

Most people tell me that around Day 8, they feel like a veil has lifted, revealing a whole new level of energy and clarity that they didn't know was possible. They feel better than they have in years, maybe decades. The headaches and stiffness go away. They think clearly. They just feel GOOD. Everyone I've watched go through this says it was totally worth toughing it out through that first week to get to the amazing feeling on the other side.

So as you start feeling those withdrawal symptoms, don't quit! Take it easy on yourself. Don't make any big plans. If you can stay home for a few days, that will help. And it is 100% okay to take over-the-counter pain relievers for your headaches just to get you through.

Remember, this short-term discomfort is going to pay off big-time.

You are strong, Rebel. I believe in you.

## WHAT'S THE DEAL WITH DETOX?

You might have heard all sorts of talk about detoxing. It's all part of the fad diet marketing machine. There's so much confusing information out there, and you might not know what to believe. And I totally get it. It's incredibly confusing. A lot of that information is designed to sell you something. So let me just break it down into simple language.

Your body already knows how to detox itself. It knows how to completely heal and cleanse itself. It just needs a few basic things from you. First of all, it needs a lot of water. I'm not talking about LaCroix or sugar-free Crystal Light or beverages made with water. No. Just plain old water with maybe some lemon or lime added for flavor. You can also add a high-quality salt to your water. Give your body lots of water, and it will naturally flush your system of any toxicity.

Also get some extra sleep if you can. Sleep is when your body does its best healing, and extra sleep may help it flush those toxins out faster.

## KEEP INGREDIENTS TO A MINIMUM

As I said earlier, if you can keep your meals to just a few ingredients, you're going to have better results. The more complicated a recipe is, the easier it is to lose track of how much you're actually consuming.

"Diet books" will give you a huge list of approved recipes and meal plans. I'm not going to do much of that. This next section will give you some ideas, but remember—YOU'RE THE BOSS. You are taking your life back, which means you are in control. You get to eat what you like. If you hate yogurt, don't eat it! This isn't a diet.

Some people need lots of variety. Some people can eat the same meal over and over again. Either way is fine. It's up to you.

Some people are recipe followers. Some people wing it. Some are happy just to eat tuna out of a can.

Whichever kind of person you are, that's perfect! Realize that you can change back and forth, too. Maybe you eat tuna six days a week, and then decide to create an amazing gourmet meal on Saturday. It's your life—take it back.

## MEAL PLAN AND PREP

It doesn't matter whether you're a parent, grandparent, or single executive on the go, we all have busy lives. One of the best things you can do to ensure your success is to plan your meals in advance. Decisions take energy, and meal planning takes one more decision off your plate for the rest of the week.

At the very least, take 10 minutes and jot down what you think you'd like to eat for dinner all week. You can always change your mind later. This gives you a starting point. If you want to, you can add breakfast and lunch to your plan. Many of my clients simply have cream in their coffee and are good until lunchtime when they just have something simple packed for work.

At the other end of the spectrum is food prepping. Some people love spending a Sunday afternoon doing all the shopping and prep work (especially chopping veggies) for the week. If that's you, great! You can get most of your lunches bagged and your dinners ready for the oven within a short, condensed time. Other people, though, find that if they prep all the food for the week, it just gets eaten faster. Go with what makes you happy and makes your busy week easier.

## GET A FEW GOOD APPLIANCES

I don't cook. My husband, Miles, does that for our household, but Code Red Rebels from all over swear by a few key appliances, like an Instant Pot and an air fryer. Ninja and immersion blenders can come in handy, too.

Some of my clients find that as they get rid of their toasters and panini presses, they can reward themselves with new appliances that help them keep to the Code Red Lifestyle.

## PREPARE FALLBACK MEALS

Even the best-laid meal plans can get tossed aside by a late meeting or soccer game. It's great to have approved meals that are already prepared, so you can grab them instead of fast food or a frozen pizza. Freezing your leftovers can even do in a pinch.

Keep simple emergency foods with you at all times. Things like nuts, beef sticks, and nut butter packets can save you from caving to a craving if you forget to bring your prepped meal.

## DITCH THE WORKAROUNDS

A few years ago, one of my custom program clients discovered the existence of microwaveable, flavored pork rinds. She immediately got in her car and spent two hours driving from supermarket to supermarket in search of these pork rinds (which she never did find). It was clear why she was struggling with her weight loss journey. She wanted what I call the workaround. It's where you go out of your way to find or create Code Red-approved versions of foods we normally avoid in weight loss mode.

I remember thinking, *If she'd just devote all that time and energy into following her custom program, instead of scouring supermarkets for pork rinds, she'd already have her weight off.*

Listen, I get that avoiding your favorite foods isn't easy. Eating is an intimate experience for most people. We develop emotional attachments to our food. It's totally normal. Even so, devoting all your time and energy into recreating foods that you're emotionally attached to, instead of just following the program, is a very slippery slope (especially in weight loss mode).

Food is fuel, not a punishment, or a reward, or a way to feel better. Eat foods you enjoy that are also approved for weight-loss mode. Ditch the workarounds. Your weight will come off faster, and once your weight is off, you can experiment with foods to find what works for you long-term. If you feel yourself about to go off the deep end and sabotage your efforts, remember to Stop, Drop, and Roll.

Now, you don't want to go out of your way looking for workarounds for a Snicker's bar, but there are some pretty major foods you're going to be taking completely out of your diet. There are perfectly reasonable substitutes that will leave you feeling satisfied *and* on plan.

## HOW TO REPLACE BREAD FOR SANDWICHES, BURGERS, AND PIZZA

Bread isn't as tough to give up when you know how to make your favorite foods without it. So here are some ideas to help you out.

HOT SANDWICHES: Just heat up the ingredients and make a "skillet" instead of a sandwich. This is especially yummy for reubens.

COLD SANDWICHES AND BURGERS: Make a lettuce wrap instead. Use a large, soft-leaf lettuce like Boston Bibb or the top half of a romaine leaf for the bread replacement. You can do a top and bottom leaf, or make a rollup. I love making BLTs (bacon, lettuce, and tomato sandwiches) this way. Many restaurants will happily give you a lettuce-wrapped burger. You won't even miss the bun.

You can also make an "inside-out" sandwich by using the meat as the outer layer, adding some mayo or guacamole and veggies, then rolling it up!

PIZZA: This is a tough one, but recipe creators have been working tirelessly to perfect the grain-free pizza crust. These are usually made from grated cauliflower and cheese, so you might want to wait until maintenance mode to try this. But you can also make mini "pizza cups" to satisfy that pepperoni craving. Put large pepperoni slices into a greased muffin tin. Add a teaspoon of sugar-free marinara and maybe an olive or grated mushroom. Bake them in the oven for a few minutes—yum!

CLOUD BREAD: Remember that I don't cook, okay? This recipe is a favorite in the high-fat, low-carb community, but it can be tricky to get just right. It's basically a bread substitute using eggs and cream of tartar (not tartar sauce!). You can find lots of recipes for cloud bread online. I also include one in the Code Red Cookbook.

## HOW TO REPLACE PASTA AND RICE

What is pasta, really? It doesn't taste like anything on its own. For most of us, it's just a vehicle for all that yummy sauce. There are some really great pasta alternatives that let you enjoy your pesto or marinara sauce as much or more than you used to.

ZUCCHINI NOODLES (AKA ZOODLES): Make long, spaghetti-like strands using a spiralizer or julienne vegetable peeler. These can be cooked or eaten raw. They make a great cold pasta salad!

SPAGHETTI SQUASH: The inside of this squash looks just like spaghetti. (Clever name, huh?) Once it's baked, you just use a fork to separate the strands. Be careful to let it cool a bit first. Those suckers are hot!

CAULIFLOWER RICE: If you're making a stir-fry or craving Chinese food, grated cauliflower makes a great substitute. It's a versatile veggie that easily takes on the flavors of the sauces or spices it's cooked with. You can use a food processor or just a regular old cheese grater to get the right consistency. Watch your fingers! You can also buy cauliflower that's already riced. Check the frozen veggies section of your supermarket.

MEAT: What? Use meat as a substitute for pasta? Well, why not? Try adding that basil pesto to a nice piece of salmon or shrimp. Skip the noodles and enjoy simple, homemade meatballs with marinara sauce and veggies. You might discover you never needed pasta in the first place.

So what should you eat in weight-loss mode? Here are some tried-and-true Rebel meal plans you might choose.

## BREAKFAST IDEAS

Please don't get hung up on breakfast foods for breakfast. Be a Rebel! If you want to eat leftover steak or a big tuna salad for your first meal of the day, awesome. If you are happy with just black coffee until noon, great. Don't eat if you're not hungry.

People always ask me for breakfast ideas, though. So here goes.

- Avocados
- Bacon
- Berries (raw or in a real-food smoothie)
- Cloud bread with cream cheese
- Eggs
- Greek yogurt (full-fat, unsweetened)
- Mini-quiche
- Omelet
- Sausage
- Code Red Pancakes
- Noatmeal

## LUNCH IDEAS

Lunch can be your main meal for the day, or it can just be something quick to tide you over until your final meal of the day. Remember you'll probably be eating that last meal much earlier than you're used to.

- Almond butter on celery
- Berries (fresh or frozen, or in a real-food smoothie)
- Bunless burger
- Inside-out sandwiches (meat rollups)
- Beef sticks
- Lettuce wraps
- Oven-roasted veggies
- Salad with or without meat
- Meat or fish (any you like)
- Veggies dipped in sour cream or Greek yogurt

## DINNER IDEAS

You are eating before 6:30, right? Keep it simple. Just pick a meat, a fat, and a vegetable. Don't make dinner into a big production, unless you really enjoy cooking.

Beware of pre-packaged meats like meatballs, sausages, and crabmeat.

Sometimes companies add grain-based fillers to make the food cheaper to produce.

- ANY MEAT: Beef, chicken, crab, fish, lobster, pork, shrimp
- ANY APPROVED VEGETABLE: Raw, roasted, or steamed; keep sauces and dressings to a minimum (but feel free to add seasonings for flavor!)
- FAJITA ROLL UPS: Flat steaks with peppers and onions rolled up inside
- "SPAGHETTI": Use one of the pasta substitutes with a sugar-free meat and marinara sauce.
- PULLED PORK: Who doesn't love pork barbecue? It takes a good 12–16 hours to slow-cook pulled pork properly. So plan ahead! And skip the ketchup-based sauce and go for the Eastern Carolina sauce; it's just vinegar and red pepper.
- MEATLOAF AND MASHED "POTATOES": Swap out those breadcrumbs for ground pork rinds and you're good. Go easy on the ketchup. And mash up some lightly steamed cauliflower instead of potatoes. Tasty!
- CHICKEN SALAD: Just mix up some chopped chicken breast with mayo and celery. Add salt and pepper and serve. So fast and easy.
- SALAD: Add some chicken or steak to your favorite salad vegetables. Presto!
- LETTUCE TACOS: Include everything but the shell. Brown some ground beef with spices. Spoon it into lettuce leaves with a little salsa and full-fat sour cream.

## SNACK IDEAS

Water! Seriously, you don't need to snack. Snacks will slow, or even stall, your weight loss. Plus, ain't nobody gonna die from skipping a meal (or a snack)!

Drinking more water can help you get over your urge to munch on something. Add some approved berries or lemon slices to your water (don't eat them - they're just for flavor). Chew sugar-free gum (so long as it doesn't bother you), or sip tea. I'm talking about tea made from a teabag, not powdered tea. There are some delicious tea flavors out there!

If the urge to snack hits in the evening, stay out of the kitchen. Go to bed early if you can.

The "three meals and two snacks a day" myth didn't work for you before, remember? It's not going to work now!

## SUNDAYS ARE FOR BRAIN PREP

In health and fitness circles, Sundays have always been meal-prep days. People use that precious time off to cook up their bacon, broccoli, chicken, or whatever they are eating consistently, so they're organized for the week. It's a great way to get yourself ahead of your food.

What about brain prep? What do you do to get your mind ready for the upcoming week?

You might think it's silly, but sticking to a food plan and making healthy decisions all day can be mentally exhausting. What you tell yourself leading up to a new week will impact how that week goes. Think about how you get yourself into the right mindset on Sunday.

Some people dread Mondays enough that Sunday is a bummer, too. "I don't want Sunday to end, I don't want to go back to work," they moan. Or if you're a parent, maybe your kids have soccer matches out of town, or late practices that you're dreading. Maybe you are in a difficult relationship, or dealing with an aging parent. I don't know what you're facing, but think about where your head is on Sunday. I call it borrowing trouble. You're worrying yourself sick over things that haven't even happened yet. Don't borrow trouble. Just take one thing at a time when it happens.

What I suggest is spend some time on Sunday planning out how you want your week to go. I'm not saying sit on a mat and meditate. I am saying envision the upcoming week on your terms. Remember, your words have power. Tell yourself that your week is going to go well.

Stand in front of your mirror and tell yourself that your weight is still going down, that your body is healing a bit more every day. Focus your attention on gratitude for everything you have, and everything that is going well. Tell yourself that you're beautiful, and that you're excellent at what you do. Use Sunday as a day to front-load positivity into your week. Talk yourself up, and visualize yourself where you want to be.

You are taking your life back and people see what you do. It's spreading to your family, your friends and coworkers. Think about how your success will influence countless other people to improve their lives and the lives of their children. It is okay to want good things and to want big things for yourself. Start your brain prep for the week on Sunday and live it out the rest of the week. Plan for your success.

## TROUBLESHOOTING IN WEIGHT-LOSS MODE

What if you're doing everything right, but you're not losing weight?

First of all, realize that when you weigh yourself every day, it's easy to think 3 or 4 days with no weight loss is a stall. Technically a stall is when you have at least one full week with no progress. Cut yourself some slack. Sometimes your body just needs to catch up with your losses so far.

Your weight is going to fluctuate, no matter what. Most days it will go down, but you may see days where it stays the same, or even goes up.

The overall trend is what we look at. At the end of the week, if you've lost five pounds, that's great! Maybe one or two days that week, your weight stayed the same, or even went up.

But at the end of the week, you're still down five pounds. Celebrate that!

Weight loss stalls can happen, so let's talk about how long you should wait before diagnosing a weight gain.

1st day > Let it go.

2nd day > Start asking questions.

3rd day > It's time to figure it out.

Here's how to figure out what's going on with your body. Just ask yourself these questions:

DID YOU GET ENOUGH SLEEP? Your body will not let go of fat if you're not getting enough sleep. Remember, sleep is the #1 rule in weight loss. If you ain't sleeping, you ain't losing.

DID YOU DRINK ALL YOUR WATER? Ice cubes don't count; you can't measure them. You really do need to drink that gallon every day, and not be drinking it up until bedtime. It makes a difference.

ARE YOU MEASURING ACCURATELY, OR ARE YOU EYE-BALL-ING IT? Do not free-pour the cream into your coffee. A heaping teaspoon is not a teaspoon—you have to level it off. Sloppy measuring is often the cause of a gain or a stall.

## SOMETIMES YOU DO EVERYTHING RIGHT AND STILL GET STUCK

It happens to everybody at some point. Say you have been drinking your water, avoiding the foods from the Do Not Eat list, keeping your sugars and carbs low, and getting your sleep.

You're doing everything you need to do, but you hop on the scale, and day after day, it doesn't budge. It's frustrating, I know. This is not the time to give up. If you stick to the program, that needle will move. If you are doing what you need to do, the weight will come off.

If your basal metabolic rate is 2,000 calories a day and you are eating 1,500 calories a day, it is physiologically impossible for your weight not to drop off. The last thing I want you to do is worry because the scale hasn't dropped.

The scale isn't the only metric you can use to track your progress. If you are eating the right things, drinking your water, and getting enough sleep, you're healing your body from the inside. Losing weight isn't the only result of your efforts. There is so much more going on than what shows up on the scale.

You're getting your energy back. Your skin and nails are finally getting what they need to grow and shine. Your cholesterol is going down. If you're working your way out of a diabetic or pre-diabetic state, your body is working hard to repair itself.

Even when the scale isn't going down, you probably notice that your clothes fit better, or are starting to feel a little loose. Trust the system. If the scale freezes, it doesn't mean that you're not still improving your health. That weight will begin to drop off again.

If custom program clients are stuck at the same weight for a full week, then my Certified Coaches and I talk with them about it. We'll help them investigate some of the different things that might be going on.

It could be their body is taking that time to really repair itself, or maybe we need to think about changing some parts of the program to account for undiagnosed food sensitivities. Either way, if that scale gets stuck, don't panic, and whatever you do, DON'T GIVE UP.

Also remember that your body didn't gain this weight and get sick overnight. Years of damage and weight gain aren't gonna reverse overnight. Trust the process, believe that your body is doing its best (because it is), and that scale will eventually start moving down again.

On the other hand, if you're not following the rules...

Be honest with yourself.

Keri Myklebust
Lewiston, Idaho
Age 45
Lost 75 pounds in 7 months and 124 total inches

I used to be an active, bubbly person. I was outgoing and constantly pushing myself. I was a little heavy in high school, but not obese by any means, but in 2016, I suffered a back injury, which left me in horrible pain. In the blink of an eye, I went from a lifetime of being extremely active to becoming almost completely sedentary.

My body could no longer do what I wanted it to and it made me miserable. I hit an all-time low and went down a path I never imagined, turning to alcohol, food and prescription medication to cope with the pain. All the weight I was gaining only added to my stress.

Even before my back injury, I'd been on a heightened health alert. My doctors were tracking several suspicious areas they thought might be cancer. I spent years waiting to hear horrible news. Doctors saw me constantly for intestinal issues, sinus infections, thyroid nodules, and skin sores. I was born premature and assumed all these problems were related to that.

**I had no idea my food choices could be factors.**

I can't even say how many different programs or diets I tried. It's embarrassing to think how many thousands of dollars I spent on programs like Ideal Protein, Weight Watchers, NutriSystem, Plexus, Shakeology, Paleo, and even tea burners. I lost weight on every single one, only to gain it back a few months later. I failed because none of them taught me what proper nutrition looks like or how to change my eating habits.

We lived in a three-story house, and there were days I could barely make it up the stairs—sometimes I even had to crawl. Realizing this would never work, my family sold the house and bought one that was mostly one level. It had a view, so at least I could see out, even when I couldn't spend time outdoors like I used to.

In the summer of 2017, we planned a family ski trip. Though I knew I wouldn't be able to get on the slopes, I took my gear anyway so my family wouldn't notice and decide to cancel the trip. I ended up spending all three days pretending to be happy as I sat in the lodge waving at skiers. I was watching my family's lives go by without me taking part.

I knew something had to change.

Soon after, I saw a friend's Facebook post about her weight melting away in a matter of months. That was the first time I heard about Cristy and the Code Red Lifestyle. By then I was desperate, so it gave me hope. I checked it out quietly because I didn't want people to know I had decided to get the weight off. This was to avoid the doubters I'd likely encounter.

I ordered *The Code Red Revolution*. Once it arrived, I read it through twice in one night. Other methods I'd tried didn't talk about the significance of water, sleep, or setting healthy boundaries—Cristy is all about that! She backed up everything with stats. There was no reason not to believe her. I was over-the-top excited about what I read and jumped in with both feet, starting the very next day.

The first week, I went through an awful detox. My head pounded and I felt horribly sick. I craved the bad foods that I had been eating for so many years. It was hard to get all my water in. But at the end of the week, I was rewarded with an eight-pound loss! My skin started to clear up and was just kind of glowing, and I started to sleep better.

Within just one week, I was completely hooked.

Adjusting to a new way of thinking was a challenge. Like wrapping my head around the idea that I should eat only when I was hungry and not at the three traditional meal times. I think the hardest part was convincing my family and friends that it was okay for me to eat like this and adjust my schedule.

I immersed myself completely. Once I got through detox, I felt incredible. There was no turning back. It felt amazing to be able to walk away from the prescription pain meds, unhealthy food, and alcohol. I hadn't felt so good in 25 years.

After I had been on the program for a while and lost 28 pounds, I attended a Code Red event. Meeting Cristy in person blew my mind! As she spoke about her lifestyle, it changed me. It all made sense and consumed me in a positive way. She gave me hope.

The Code Red lifestyle began to heal my emotions too, benefiting my mind, body, and spirit. Knowing that I'm in full control of my life feels amazing.

My biggest struggle in the beginning was having people judge me, waiting for me to fail. This program's community and the support of friends and family gave me the drive to continue.

I believe 100% in this lifestyle and its many benefits. My mind has had a chance to heal itself. I'm not going to let it go back to the way it was before.

When I started the program, my initial milestone weight was 170 pounds, and I hit that fairly quickly. Soon I hit 160 and—all of a sudden—I was in the 150s. I just started crying. In the military, I weighed 145 pounds, and I never thought I'd see that weight ever again...*but I got there.* The cool part is I could drop another 10 pounds if I wanted to. I'd never experienced this kind of control before.

The scale victory is one thing, but my non-scale victories were even more rewarding.

In April of 2018, just four months into this new lifestyle, I had my annual mammogram. They didn't detect any new issues. What's more, a previous area of concern hadn't grown at all and did not require another biopsy. I can't even tell you the joy and the relief I experienced, after so many years of uncertainty.

Before Code Red, one of my doctors discovered that my thyroid was enlarged. Thankfully, the biopsy identified it as non-cancerous, but the doctor said if it was still enlarged after six months it would need to be removed.

At the follow-up, my doctor could hardly believe my weight loss and said I was almost unrecognizable. As he was dancing around the room in celebration, I could barely breathe while waiting for him to check my thyroid. I was afraid of what he would find.

Finally, he said, "Keri, your thyroid has shrunk." There was no need for surgery. When I got to my car I just started bawling, so overwhelmed with happiness. I called my mom and could hardly get the words out.

The weight loss reduced my debilitating back pain. My skin has healed, the intestinal issues and sinus infections are gone and I can fit into any chair, airplane seat, or amusement park ride. I have to say, for anybody who hasn't been able to do those things, it feels wonderful when you can.

The first time I wrapped a hotel towel all the way around me, I just started laughing. Now I can pull anything out of my closet to wear, knowing it will fit and fit well. I know I'll feel confident in whatever I choose.

I have more energy than I could have imagined. I can hike with my family. I can bike and kayak. I can *use* my body again. The best part is that when I am out with my family, I'm 100% with them—no more sitting on the sidelines.

I was surprised to see the people around me change their lives after watching me change mine. My husband joined in with me after he read the book and our daughter followed next. That was particularly exciting because we had taught our kids so many bad habits around food and eating through the years. Seeing my daughter's happiness and success gives me so much joy.

In addition, my 70-year-old mom, my mother-in-law, my friends—all of them tried the lifestyle and enjoyed the results. I love that I get to be a positive example to anyone who might run into me. The ripple effect keeps me fueled.

This lifestyle is definitely a revolution and it's catching on. So many people have taken their lives back with Code Red! Some only needed to lose 10 pounds, others needed to lose 200 or more. They all questioned it at first, they had all tried other diets. They all had doubts. Every single one of them succeeded. The only regret I ever hear is that they waited too long to try it.

**That's my advice to anyone who's curious about it: Don't wait. This lifestyle will change your life for the better, so quickly and in such a profound way.**

I know what it's like to live overweight. You're out there and you're heavy, you hurt and you don't want to be noticed. You avoid putting yourself out in front of people because you lack the confidence. It doesn't have to be that way.

You have the power to change the way you look and feel. You can build more confidence than you've ever thought possible. All you have to do is want it enough.

The Code Red Lifestyle will get you there. Your mental state, your physical state—everything is going to improve. Just give it a chance.

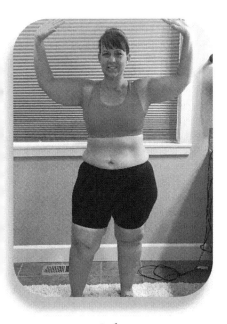

*Before*

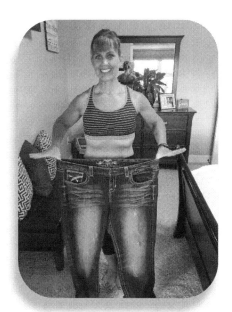

*After*

# CHAPTER 8

# MAKING IT STICK: HOW TO MAINTAIN YOUR WEIGHT LOSS FOREVER

L ET'S FACE IT—ANYBODY can lose weight.

But can you keep it off for the rest of your life? That's the key question.

A terrifying statistic says over two-thirds of people who lose weight gain it back again. That's usually because they used a quick fix or a gimmick or a crap-ton of exercise to lose it in the first place. It's not sustainable. I want to encourage you—maintaining your goal weight is not difficult. We haven't come all this way to have you gain it all back in a year. Even if you've done exactly that in the past—*especially* if you've done that in the past.

All you have to do is keep following three rules for maintaining your weight loss:

- Step on the scale every day.
- Keep drinking your water.
- Keep junk food out of your house.

## STAY ON THAT SCALE

You have to keep weighing yourself. Not because the scale is the end-all and be-all. Not because that's the only way to measure good health—it's not. But that scale is your first line of defense. Get on that scale every single morning, because if it says you're 2 pounds up, that's going to be your first indication that you are off track. What's 2 pounds?

Well, that 2 pounds turns into 4, and that 4 turns into 6, and that 6 will turn into 10. Pretty soon, you're back to being 30, 40, or 50 pounds overweight. That scale is going to keep your desired weight right in the forefront of your mind so you can get back on track before that 2 pounds becomes 10 or 20 and you're back to square one.

Get on that scale, every single morning.

## KEEP DRINKING YOUR WATER

Whatever amount of water you drank to get your weight down, you must keep drinking that amount. It's imperative. When you're dehydrated, your body sends signals that it's hungry. Truth is, your body's not really hungry, it's thirsty. If you stay well-hydrated, you'll feel full. You'll have energy, you'll stay focused, and you'll even sleep better. So many good things happen when you drink water. Keep drinking!

## KEEP YOUR HOUSE A SAFE ZONE

Never, and I mean *never,* allow junk food back into your house. There are times when junk food will sneak in, perhaps for a party, or a guest will bring it with them. You've got to get rid of it in less than 24 hours. The longer junk food stays in your house the greater the chance that you will eat it. You don't need to do that. Willpower eventually runs out, and that absolutely cannot happen. You can never allow junk food to stay in your house.

You are amazing.

You deserve to live a long and healthy life. Backsliding is not going to happen—not this time.

These rules help keep you accountable to yourself and your goal. If you know how much you weigh every day, you will be less likely to swing by Dunkin' Donuts for a croissant. If you are drinking a gallon of water every day, you'll feel too full to crave a snack you know you don't need. When you get home and still want a snack, you'll have healthier options if you've kept the junk out of your house.

## TRANSITIONING TO MAINTENANCE: HOW TO ADD FOODS BACK IN

You've made it! After months of following the process and being extremely good to your body, you have finally reached your goal weight. You're excited, and you want to go out and celebrate.

What do you do? How do you add back the foods we avoid in weight loss mode?

I can't stress enough that you should not reward yourself with food. When you've reached your goal weight, take a trip across the country to see your best friend from college, or buy yourself that cute dress you have been eyeing for months. You should reward yourself, because you have worked awfully hard to get where you are now. But don't do it with food.

That being said, you might be asking yourself, "Well, Cristy, what about those foods you said we could eat again after we reached our goal weight?" Here's how Rebels handle that.

## START SLOWLY

I'll talk about specific foods in a moment., but this is key: You've got to start slow when you're adding food back in. Fruit, for example, is a great food to start with, but not by inhaling a fruit salad. Instead, start with one piece of fruit a day. The reason for this is your own comfort. If you reach your goal weight and then eat two apples, a banana and a cup of brown rice in one day, you don't know how your body is going to react to those foods being reintroduced. You could bloat, your stomach might cramp, or your joints could ache.

For example, I know that I cannot metabolize beans. Beans are a great maintenance food, with plenty of protein and fiber, but I simply can't eat them. You may find foods that your body just doesn't want to work with and you will have an easier time identifying those foods if you pick one from the list per day to try. That way, if your body does react poorly, you will know what caused it.

## BE STRATEGIC

Reintroducing foods will work for the rest of your life, but only if you're strategic about it.

It's important to take your time, reintroduce one food at a time, and see how your body reacts.

If you see a gain on the scale the next day, wait until your weight returns to goal before you reintroduce a new food. Otherwise, you could pack on a bunch of the weight you lost.

Take it slowly and methodically. Pay attention not only to the scale, but to how your body responds. This is how you'll find what works for you.

## PLAN INDULGENCES

You may have heard of the 90/10 method. It's where you eat clean 90% of the time, and eat from the foods-to-avoid side of the Code Red foods list 10% of the time.

I call that 10% a planned indulgence.

That's right - I want you to plan your indulgences.

Say you are meeting a friend on Saturday night and that is going to be your planned indulgence.

Follow the Code Red process exactly all week long. Get in your full gallon of water, eat your fat, veggies, and protein all week, and get the sleep you need every night. Do that Sunday through Saturday afternoon, and then Saturday night, you enjoy your planned indulgence. The next morning, you are right back to drinking your water and eating clean.

If you follow this process, the occasional indulgence is okay. If you are eating clean the rest of the time, you will be fine. One meal is not enough to derail six and a half days of clean nutrition.

One thing to be aware of, however, is you may not enjoy that indulgence food when you do get it. It may not taste as great as you remember, or your body may have a reaction. I know I seldom feel good after going back to processed food.

Bottom line: If you are eating clean 90% of the time, you can eat off-plan 10%, but know that it might not agree with you. Know that, especially if you have a weight gain or other reaction, you return to clean Code Red eating the rest of the time.

## DRAW YOUR LINE IN THE SAND

This is it. This next paragraph is how you're going to stay at a healthy weight for the rest of your life! Are you ready?

Pick a number that's two or three pounds (no more than five) above your goal weight. That's your line in the sand. That is THE NUMBER YOU WILL NOT CROSS. Got it?

Okay, now when you weigh yourself every day, the second your weight goes above that, you hop right back into weight-loss mode until you lose back down to your goal. Chances are, you've caught it soon enough that it will only take a few days to get that number back down.

Simple, huh?

This strategy has helped my clients keep their weight off for years. They don't even have to think about it anymore. They can go on vacation and indulge. Then when they get home, they hop back to the weight-loss rules and any excess weight is gone in no time.

No stress. No blame. No guilt. No fear. You're such a Rebel!

## STAYING POWER: STICKING TO YOUR NEW WAY OF THINKING

Let's talk about staying motivated.

The time of year when people are most motivated is New Year's Day, right? So many people make those whole-hearted resolutions. Let's face it, after the ball drops, a lot of people drop their motivation, too.

Anyone can stick with something new for the first two weeks of the new year. I know you can hit the gym five times a week...for the first two weeks. How do you keep going long after you feel like doing it? How do you stay motivated?

Here are three tips for staying motivated long after those warm fuzzy feelings are gone—no matter what time of year it is.

1.  **Clean Out Your Social Feed.** No matter how you spin it, social media is a part of our lives. We're on our favorite platforms con-

tinuously. So get rid of the crap that doesn't line up with your new way of thinking. For example, if you're trying to cut back on wine, stop following sites that talk about wine.

You know what I mean. Advertisements, or worse, friends' posts that say things like "It's wine-thirty" or "I need a glass of wine" or "Who wants to meet up for a glass of wine?"

You don't need that feeding into your thoughts. If you're trying to cut back on eating sweets, you don't need a bunch of dessert recipes in your newsfeed. You don't need to read posts about how to bake the perfect chocolate cake or Grandma's chocolate chip cookies. Cleaning out your newsfeed will help you clean out your body and your mind.

2.  **Hang Out With Like-Minded People.** The old saying goes, "Show me your friends and I'll show you your future." That's exactly right. If you're trying to get healthy, find people who, like you, are motivated to get to bed early so they can get all their sleep. Go to breakfast with them, have coffee with them. Spend time absorbing their mindsets and habits. Hang out with people that are like-minded.

3.  **Buy Some High-Quality Clothes That Fit.** It sounds kind of simple, I know, but go out and get some good-quality, nice-fitting clothes. As you lose weight, your jeans will get droopy and start to fall off. Your shirts will start to look like dresses. At first, you'll be excited. It means you're making progress, but you'll quickly find that those baggy clothes just make you feel frumpy. Loose pants can even make you feel like you could eat a little more.

When your clothes fit properly, you feel amazing! People notice your progress and you're less likely to stray off the plan when you know how awesome you look.

If you're worried about having to replace your whole wardrobe every few weeks (yes, it does happen that fast), you can always shop at thrift stores. Or do a clothing swap with a friend who is just a little bit ahead of you. You don't have to spend a lot of money, but the investment is so worth it. You're worth it!

When you reach your goal weight, spring for those quality clothes that fit - for all the reasons above, but also because they make a great non-food reward!

Leisha Pielak
California
Age 30
Lost 115 pounds

I'd been obese since I was very young. I vividly remember always being the biggest kid in class. I remember being 9 years old, lying in the bathtub wondering why I was so much bigger than all the other kids. I remember visualizing a doctor slicing off my fat rolls.

Throughout my teens and into my 20s, I continued gaining weight, despite playing sports and staying active. It got to the point where I couldn't look at myself in the mirror without tearing myself down inch by inch.

I couldn't even bend over far enough to tie my own shoes without completely cutting off my airway. I had to loosely pre-tie my shoes, drop them on the floor, and wiggle my feet in to get them on—I contemplated buying a shoe horn.

In 2016, my husband and I bought a Toyota Tacoma and I was so excited. Our growing family moved and traveled a lot—we needed that pickup. Yet the first time I sat in the driver's seat, I was devastated. I couldn't buckle the seatbelt. The buckle dug into my side, it was too painful to drive.

I was too ashamed to tell my husband. Can you imagine? "Hey, by the way, babe, I'm too fat to drive the truck. Can you take me?"

Of course, I constantly tried to lose weight. I tried everything. If a program said it could help me lose weight, I was in. Probably the most dangerous thing I ever tried was HCG drops mixed with phentermine while working out two hours a day and not eating. (Literally deadly!)

In two months I had lost about 50 pounds, but I'd always gain it all back as soon as I resumed eating and stopped working out. My husband was away at tech school during this time, so I was living at my mother-in-law's house. I would wake up really early, go to the gym for at least two hours and come home.

Nancy, my mother-in-law would ask, "What are you eating today?" And I'd say, "Oh, I'll eat something," but she knew full well I wasn't going to eat that day. I often went several days at a time without eating anything. The HCG drops suggested a 500-calorie limit, and I thought staying under that would help me lose weight faster. Nancy would make me protein shakes and watch me drink them to make sure I ate.

I avoided seeing the doctor, because I hated hearing the "You need to lose weight" speech, complete with handfuls of pamphlets, lists of local gyms, diet foods, and a number for a nutritionist. After those appointments, all I wanted to do was go home and drown myself in food. I'd grab a large spoon from my drawer and say, "What if I just have one? It's only from a spoon, so it doesn't really count."

It's easy to lose count when you don't count.

Extra bowls of cereal and extra bites of ice cream from the freezer. I epitomized food addiction, always thinking about what to eat next. Looking back, I had been at rock bottom my entire life. I didn't know what anything else felt like. So when a little glimmer of hope shined my way, I grabbed it.

I heard about Code Red in 2017 through my mother-in-law at our yearly Christmas get-together. She mentioned it a few times over the visit, but didn't really push it. By that time I'd become so desperate to lose weight, I'd settled on bariatric surgery. I had a referral from my doctor and was ready to meet with a surgeon.

Once back home, Nancy called and Code Red came up in the conversation again.

She told me about the 10 Pound Takedown Challenge and said she wanted us to do it together. Having tried so many different things, I was skeptical. How could this be any different? Nancy told me one of her best friends had lost a bunch of weight with Code Red and felt amazing.

I resisted, not wanting to throw money away on another weight-loss attempt. Nancy offered to pay for my challenge, provided I agree to go all in for the duration. Since it wasn't my $47 being flushed down the toilet, I agreed.

Then I got a look at Cristy—this amazing, intense, successful woman with a colorful mohawk—that piqued my interest, being a mohawk fan myself.

Despite my skepticism, that challenge changed everything. I lost 12 pounds in just over two weeks. Nothing had ever worked like that before. I used part of our tax refund to purchase a custom program before the challenge ended.

**It's the best decision I've ever made.**

Code Red stood out because I could lose weight without feeling hungry and I didn't have to exercise. I mean, what magic is this? Plus I was encouraged to eat delicious foods! I ate bacon, avocado, cucumbers, and ranch dressing every single day for about 12 months and lost all that weight. What other program can do that for you?

Rethinking dinner was a struggle. Big dinners were our thing—hefty plates of pasta or rice, meat and potatoes. I'd think about dinner all day. Then, eating dinner, I'd start thinking about what I would eat the next day. It was an obsession.

Being a military family, any time we had out-of-town guests, we'd show them all of our favorite places. Before Code Red, all of those were restaurants. We'd take our guests to our favorite sandwich shops, or the breakfast cafes with the best pancakes. After Code Red, all that ended. It was an adjustment to host our guests without the entire visit revolving around the next meal. We save hundreds of dollars because we aren't constantly going out to eat.

One thing Cristy says that really stuck with me is, "Ain't nobody getting out of the rules." All it takes is one slip-up. That one slip-up won't put all that weight back on., but when you justify "just one" chip, that leads to "just one more" chip—before long, the bag is empty. That leads to a cycle of guilt and shame, and that is what will derail you.

I did not allow myself one chip. I refused to throw that sugary-junk creamer in my coffee—not even once. I knew that while one bite wouldn't kill me or put 50 pounds back on me overnight, it would send me right back into that cycle. No chip is worth that.

Of course, my first big milestone was getting into One-derland—a weight under 200. I hadn't been under 200 pounds since 2013 when I had my son. Until Code Red, I didn't believe it was even possible.

Part of me didn't believe it would last. I remember thinking, *Tomorrow I'm going to wake up and I'm going to be 200 pounds.* But I wasn't. The next day, I was even lower, and my weight continued to drop. I haven't seen 200 since. It's amazing!

The next exciting milestone was when I dropped below 170. I hadn't seen 170 since taking that dangerous mix of HCG drops and phentermine. Reaching 170 without starving myself, using drops or pills, or exercising for two hours a day? That drove it home for me. I believed I could actually get to my goal weight. I had cried when Cristy set it, because it didn't seem like a real number. We all want to reach our goal, but part of you feels like it's never going to happen. My goal weight was less than I had weighed in junior high.

The day I reached it was incredible.

Now I'm a few pounds BELOW that weight. It's where my body likes to be and I can tell you, it IS attainable. You can get there.

I can tie my shoes now, climb the stairs, chase my kids, and do countless other things I couldn't before. Avoiding bariatric surgery was a huge blessing, but my favorite part of finding the Code Red Lifestyle™? I can comfortably drive that $30,000 pickup truck.

The idea of maintaining my weight loss was scary at first. I spent the 12 months prior to maintenance weighing, logging, and measuring every scrap of food that I ate, and suddenly I'm expected to just eyeball it? I quickly realized, however, that maintenance is more about listening to your body than focusing on amounts.

After spending so much time in weight-loss mode, I already knew which foods my body liked and disliked, when to eat during the day—I knew what it needed. If I gain a couple of pounds for whatever reason, I know exactly what I need to do to take it back off. I have the tools and I'm in charge.

Avoid rewarding yourself with food. Focus on getting the weight off and save indulgences for maintenance. Even then, it's important to plan them and to pay attention to how your body responds.

Community matters. My mother-in-law and I bought our first challenges together and we bought our custom programs together. We talked every day, sharing our stressors and our victories. We participated in our coaching group every day and developed relationships with those people and our coaches. We looked forward to the accountability coaching videos so we could celebrate our success or get help when we struggled.

Even after reaching maintenance, we stayed in our coaching groups. Hitting your goal weight isn't the end of the journey.

The other rebels become your family. If someone's struggling, the community reaches out. Being around like-minded people is essential to your success. Surround yourself with people who have the same goal as you.

**Accountability and community are everything—nobody does this alone.**

With everything we do there's a ripple effect. Your Code Red journey is no exception. You cling to the people you relate to. You hear their stories and listen to their advice.

People will watch your journey. My mother-in-law and I started doing Code Red, just the two of us. The next thing I knew, my mom and dad both joined the lifestyle. A friend of mine joined a challenge and they've all been wildly successful.

I'd been obese since childhood—I know what hopelessness feels like. It's okay to be scared—to feel whatever you're feeling. Just don't let those feelings hold you back. You deserve to be the best possible version of yourself. It will take work, but you're worth it.

I know you've tried everything else. So did I. Trust me. You have nothing to lose by trying this.

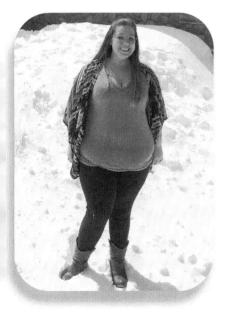

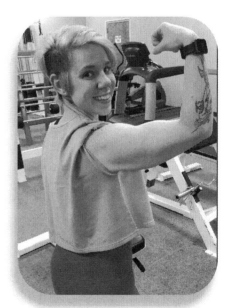

*Before*                    *After*

# CHAPTER 9

# FREE YOURSELF FROM THE WEIGHT-LOSS MYTHS

I WAS 14 THE first time I saw a muscular woman. A Miss Fitness USA competition came on one of the three channels we could watch on our old TV. I don't think they even have Miss Fitness competitions anymore, but back then they were pretty popular. My jaw dropped when I saw those women walk out on the stage.

My family lived in a tiny rural town of three thousand occupants, so there wasn't much local variety. We all looked like middle-America farmers. I could not get over how beautiful those women on the TV were. I was mesmerized. I didn't know anything about weightlifting or nutrition or anything, but I saw those muscles and I wanted them! *Somehow*, I promised myself, *I'm going to be that beautiful one day.*

So I did what I thought would get me closer to that goal—I got a job cleaning up a gym. I cleaned mats, machines, and toilets. I was basically a janitor, but in my mind, it was how I would start moving closer to fitness. As time went by, I learned how to exercise and train. After a lot of work, I became a personal trainer. More and more clients came to me to lose weight, so I did what I thought was the right thing: I helped them exercise the weight off, just like I was taught.

It sort of worked. For some people. Some of the time.

If exercise is actually the way to address a weight problem—if it's really calories in, calories out and a calorie is a calorie—surely it should work for everyone, all of the time, right? Except it didn't.

I couldn't figure out why.

The mystery continued for several years, until the day it finally happened: I got fat.

My weight gain started toward the end of my boxing career. Just a few pounds at first. No big deal, right? Except it didn't stop with just a few pounds. I kept gaining and gaining, even after I retired from boxing and took up elite-level road cycling. I was riding my road bike 300 miles a week and keeping up with the fastest men. To this day I hold cycling records that have not been broken. My husband and I took trips to Europe, where the only thing we did was ride our bikes for 70 miles every day. Here I was, training the hardest I had in my entire life and burning more calories with exercise than I ever had.

Yet I was gaining weight.

If exercise is how you address a weight problem, how could it be that I was both the fattest and the fittest I'd ever been? How could it be that my thigh fat was busting out of my skin-tight cycling shorts? How could it be that my knees were slapping into my belly fat when I pedaled? It just didn't make sense.

Determined to figure out why this was happening, I did some research. That's when I discovered the truth. The government recommendation of "eat less, exercise more" just doesn't work in the real world. You're going to blow out a knee before you even come close to working off that caramel macchiato you drank before work.

The right nutrition is the key to weight loss! It has nothing to do with exercise.

Let that sink in for a minute because you're probably shaking your head right now. *Uh-uh Cristy, you're crazy. I gotta exercise. That's my problem, I just need more exercise.* I get it. The government, your family, your friends, every magazine on the planet, your doctor—everyone has told you in one way or another that you're not losing weight because *you're not trying hard enough.* If you would just exercise more, it would all even out.

Well guess what I say to that...Bullcrap!

I've proved it over and over. I proved it with myself. I proved it with my family. Over the past few years, I've proved it with literally thousands and thousands of Rebels who finally got off the treadmill and actually lost their weight.

Now don't get me wrong, exercise is great. It's important for a whole bunch of reasons. I bike and run and move my body every day. I'm not telling you that you shouldn't exercise. I am telling you it's not going to help you lose weight. Exercise and weight loss are two separate animals! Killing yourself for hours and hours in the gym when you're overweight is not only pointless, it's downright dangerous. Your joints, your heart, your muscles—they need *appropriate levels* of exercise based on your physical condition. Got it?

This discovery not only set me free and helped me lose my weight the right way, it got me wondering what other myths were floating around out there keeping people obese and sick. Turns out there were more than I ever imagined and in this part of the book, I'm going to shine a light on the ones I see keeping people trapped as prisoners in their own bodies.

It's time to set you FREE.

It's like that movie The Matrix. You get to decide. Take the blue pill, continue on the way you have been, and stay overweight. Or take the red pill and learn the truth. Take your life back forever. I'm just going to assume you took the red pill and keep going.

Let's get started debunking the myths keeping you fat and sick.

## MYTH #1: YOU HAVE TO EXERCISE TO LOSE WEIGHT.

Let's get this out in the open right now. Exercise is a wonderful thing. It helps your mood. It keeps your circulation stable. You should absolutely exercise. I was a professional athlete and got paid to exercise.

But hear me...

**Exercise has nothing to do with losing weight.**

I know some people reading this might be mad at me. A ton of money has been spent to convince you that you have to exercise off the calories... but my experience with thousands of actual clients proves otherwise.

For so many people, exercise has become some sort of sick self-torture. They punish themselves at the gym and the more brutal the workout, the more virtuous they feel. Exercise is not a punishment. It's a glorious celebration of your physical ability. It's a thank you to your body for getting you through another day. It's a reward.

You know what else? You're not "bad" if you skip the gym in favor of an extra hour of sleep. People are far more sleep-deprived than exercise-deprived in this country. If your goal is to lose pounds, sleep will do you more good.

We have all heard that exercise is the way to address weight loss, right? But take a look behind the curtain for a minute. Who's been telling us this?

Hmm, could it be the fitness industry? Could it be the very people who stand to make billions of dollars if you believe the lies?

The whole idea is that exercise burns calories, right? So theoretically, if you exercise long enough or hard enough, you'll burn off that stored-up fat. Let me clear this up for you right now. You'll never be able to exercise enough to lose more than a couple of pounds without also managing what goes into your mouth.

You're more likely to blow out a knee before you lose any significant weight. You can exercise twice a day if you want, but if you eat a larger dinner that night or you eat a pickle with your cheeseburger, then most likely your weight will be up the next day, not down.

Exercise doesn't matter when it comes to weight loss. It's hard for me to say that, having studied exercise physiology in college. It's hard for me to say that, having made my career as a professional athlete, but it is the truth. When I was a professional trainer I would put people through grueling workouts, but they never saw the results that my nutrition clients see now.

You will never outrun your fork. You can't out-train a bad diet.

## WHEN IT IS TIME TO EXERCISE

All that being said, when the time is right, exercise is hugely beneficial. You will know when you are ready to add in exercise. Your body will tell you. You will actually want to take a walk or play with your kids in the park.

For our custom program clients, exercise happens when they have gotten down to goal weight and they want to get rid of the *jigglies*. Welcome to weight training! The good news is that anyone can lose weight and they can lose as much as they would like. However, here's another hard truth—you probably won't look really good naked unless you begin weight training. You can compare four women who are the same weight and each one might have a completely different shape. This is *body composition* and weight training is what allows you to alter yours.

When you have achieved your goal weight and begin to see the positive changes in your life from exercise, you won't believe what you can do. I hear people say all the time, "I was never able to pick up my grandchild before, but now I can!" I love stories like that, and it doesn't take fancy moves or fancy equipment. It doesn't take a gym membership; it takes consistency.

Age isn't an excuse either. People tell me, "I'm not 20 anymore." Neither am I. If you start at the beginning, listen to your body, and stay consistent every day after that, it will not matter how old you are. One of my clients is over 60 and runs full marathons. Stick to the plan, make consistency your unbreakable rule, and ENJOY YOUR EXERCISE. It's a reward, not a punishment.

## MYTH #2: YOU HAVE TO EAT LOW-FAT

"Fat is bad."

"Eating fat will kill you."

"Low-fat foods are the only ones that are healthy."

Those are the kinds of things we've been told about fat. There's all kinds of data that supposedly backs up this huge myth, but who has time to read it all? We believe what we are repeatedly told. Fat is bad. We're trying to *not be fat*, so it makes sense that we shouldn't eat it. Plus, fat makes food taste good. It's satisfying. It fills us up. So that *must* mean it's bad for us, right?

Not so fast.

We need fat to survive. It's a critical component to our human system. Yet we get confused about it because it's the same stuff hanging off our tummies and our butts that we're trying so hard to get rid of.

A lot of the confusion stems from the fact there's body fat and there's dietary fat.

They are NOT the same thing.

The fat on your body—the stuff you want to lose—that's nothing more than stored-up energy. When your body runs out of primary fuel, it will start using that stored fuel. The problem for most people is that their bodies never run out of primary fuel because they keep consuming it. So they stay overweight.

When we refer to "fat" as a nutrient, or *dietary fat*, we're looking at an amazing substance. You can't live without it. Fat helps your hair and nails grow. It assists in normal brain development and helps you absorb vitamins A, D, E, and K. You can get fat from animal products like chicken, bacon, and steak. You can also get healthy fat from plant sources like avocados, nuts, coconut oil, extra virgin olive oil, nuts, and seeds.

Government guidelines since 1977 have recommended that Americans reduce the amount of fat in their diets to avoid the risk of stroke, heart disease, and other problems. In response to the low-fat call to arms, the food industry stepped up to produce hundreds of thousands of products that they market as "healthy" and "fat-free," yet are totally devoid of nutrition. We shovel fistfuls of fat-free snacks into our mouths, not realizing we are just making ourselves fatter and less healthy.

The fat-free craze that has taken over our society is a major cause of our obesity epidemic. The government said "eat less fat," so the food industry responded with hundreds of thousands of new "healthy" products labeled low fat and fat-free. There was a major problem, though. The products tasted terrible! So the food industry figured out that they could add sugar and simple carbs back in to make it taste good and *still be fat-free* according to the label laws.

Contrary to what the government or your well-meaning neighbors might say, lowering your dietary fat intake will not make any difference in your weight loss. Adding in the right fats—like avocados, olives, and naturally occurring oils such as olive and coconut—can actually aid weight loss. (As long as you're very careful with your calorie consumption.)

Dietary fat doesn't make you fat. Sugar makes you fat.

It contains *way more* energy than you need, and excess energy is stored away.

Control how much sugar and simple carbohydrates you're consuming and you'll be well on your way to that weight loss and healthy lifestyle you desire.

## MYTH #3: I NEED THREE MEALS AND TWO SNACKS PER DAY.

In today's world we are still led to believe that three meals and two snacks a day are necessary for our survival. Allow me to let you in on a little secret—we don't need to eat that often! You don't have to starve yourself or suffer from cravings either. It's all about the chemistry. People feel like they need to eat frequently throughout the day because of the kinds of food they're eating.

Dietary fat is directly related to satiety or feeling full and content. When you strip fat away with "healthy" low-fat or fat-free foods, you lose that beautiful feeling of being satiated. So when you wake up and have a bagel or some toast for breakfast, you set yourself up for failure. You're setting the stage for cravings and hunger all day long.

In very simple terms, when you consume low-fat foods your blood sugar spikes. It makes you feel good for a little while. But in order to get that spike under control, the body releases insulin. If you're pre-diabetic or diabetic, you may need to medicate yourself to get the insulin you need.

Here's why you feel like you need to eat all day long. When blood sugar drops, you feel hungry or irritable, so you eat some crackers or a muffin to bring it back up. Then the body releases more insulin to bring it down again. Sugar spike—>insulin release—>sugar drop. You end up on a chemical rollercoaster of blood sugar levels. Where if you just ate some fat, you wouldn't feel hungry because there would be no sugar spikes.

This is not a personal attack on diabetics. This is me explaining the trap many diabetics are in without even knowing it. It's a trap I want you to avoid. These blood sugar highs and lows are most often caused by eating the wrong foods and eating them frequently.

Here's another problem with frequent eating. One of insulin's jobs is to transform extra energy into fat. So guess what? When you eat every couple of hours and have a lot of insulin floating around in your blood, you're sending the message to store fat. Store it now...store it good!

If you think about it in caveman terms, it's summer time. The eating is good. There's tons of sugar everywhere in the form of fresh fruit. You're eating a lot of it, so you can store it up as fat so you can survive through the winter when food will be scarce. Except winter never comes. You just keep storing and storing and storing.

The good news is that changing your eating habits can help you escape the hunger trap. One of my clients shared that her husband has struggled with his blood sugar since the Vietnam war ended. For 40 years his doctor has been on his case about high blood sugar. By following the Code Red Lifestyle, he was able to get his pre-diabetic state under control. By changing what and how often he eats, he wasn't hungry and avoided having to control his blood sugar through medication. This way of eating literally saved his life.

Don't be afraid of reducing your food intake to two or three times a day. If you're eating the right foods, your blood sugar will stay pretty stable. You probably won't even notice feeling hungry for a long period of time because you're not experiencing the blood sugar highs and lows that trigger cravings.

## MYTH #4: SUGAR IS OKAY IN MODERATION.

Sugar is hands-down the biggest cause of sickness, disease, and cancer in today's society. I know that's a bold statement and a lot of people get defensive when I talk about it. It has been proven time and time again. It's poison at the levels we consume it today. There's a safe sugar threshold for humans, just like there's a safe threshold of anything—even arsenic.

Across the board, nutritionists agree that we should get no more than about 25 grams of sugar per day, which is roughly 6 teaspoons. Most people consume more than that within an hour of waking up. The average American gets about 150 grams of sugar per day, which is astonishing. That's just a mind-blowing amount of sugar.

The problem is we just don't realize how often we're consuming it. Okay, yeah, that morning doughnut has sugar. That's easy to spot, but what about the healthy salad you're eating for lunch? The one with the dried cranberries (26g of sugar in 1/3 cup) and the low-fat dressing with added sugar?

Food doesn't have to taste sweet to have added sugar. In fact, as you consume more sugar, your taste buds become numb to sweetness. You have to add more and more sugar to get the same sensation of sweetness. Once you remove sugar from your diet, your taste buds return to normal and foods you used to love will suddenly be too sickly sweet to eat.

If you want to dive deep into the science behind sugar and its unholy alliance with the manufactured food industry, I highly recommend reading *Salt, Sugar, Fat* and watching the documentary *Fed Up*. Let's put all that aside for now and just focus on the effects sugar has on your weight.

Remember that your body can run on glucose or ketones. Glucose is sugar. So consuming sugar will provide energy (until the crash), but since we consume way more than we need, it gets stored away as fat. Once again, your body is just doing its job—saving up for when there's no food available.

The Code Red answer to this is pretty obvious—don't eat sugar or foods that easily break down into sugar, such as bread, pasta, or alcohol. If you're trying to burn excess fat by converting it to ketones, you can't be adding sugar to the equation.

Easier said than done, right? Sugar is everywhere!

Can you imagine a life where you have no cravings for sugary sweets or desserts? It is totally possible! When you eat a high-fat diet regularly, there are no spikes. There are no crashes. There are no physical cravings.

It's really simple to keep your sugar intake down, once you become aware of how much sugar is in everything. The food industry has gotten really tricky. They've figured out how to call sugar other names to fool you—over 61 other names. If you see words like these on your food labels, you're looking at sugar: brown sugar, cane crystals, cane sugar, corn sweetener, corn syrup, corn syrup solids, crystal dextrose, dextrose, evaporated cane juice, fructose sweetener, or fruit juice.

Sugar is cheap and it makes manufactured foods taste better—so they add tons of it to just about everything you consume.

Here's the dirty little secret about sugar: it's addictive. The more you eat it, the more you crave it. It's been proven to be 8 times more addictive than cocaine. That's not a number I just made up. It's actually been measured and proven!

Can you imagine how hard it would be to just "unplug" from cocaine or heroin using pure willpower? It would be just about impossible, especially if it was just lying around your home and you were expected to use it multiple times a day. Could anyone ever detox from drugs if they were advertised to them 24/7?

Of course not!

We demonize and vilify addictive drugs like cocaine, heroin, and even tobacco, but sugar isn't classified as a drug, even though it's just as addictive and causes horrible health problems. Sugar is celebrated in this country. In fact, it seems to be a required component of any celebration we hold—from birthdays to weddings to holidays. It's added to just about every manufactured food available. It's marketed to children through cartoons and video games. Unless you live under a rock, it's practically impossible to escape the influence of sugar. It's not your fault that you're addicted to it—you're simply part of a massive marketing campaign designed to make a few companies extremely wealthy.

Track your food for a week, and I guarantee you will be shocked by what you discover. Even when you're eating "healthy," you're probably going to find yourself way over that recommended 25g of sugar. What about natural sugars like honey, coconut sugar and raw cane sugar? Those don't count, do they?

It all counts!

Added sugars are easy to spot. If you're eating anything in a box or a wrapper, it's probably got added sugar. Fruits and vegetables have natural sugars. Honey and maple syrup are natural sugars. It all counts toward that 25g limit.

The good news is that berries like strawberries and blueberries are low-sugar. So they can be eaten during weight-loss mode. Just don't overdo it. Track everything.

No one is going to police your sugar consumption for you. In fact, manufacturers are going to do their best to get you to consume as much as possible. If it has a package, a box, or a wrapper, check the label for sugar "con"-tent. Better yet, just don't eat it at all. The less you eat out of packages, the better.

## WHAT ABOUT ALTERNATIVE SWEETENERS?

Here's a tricky subject: Is it okay to substitute alternative sweeteners when you're cutting out sugar? The answer is that *it depends*. You have to pay very close attention to what happens with your weight when you consume different types and different amounts of this stuff. Different people have different tolerances. You might be able to use monk fruit or stevia—or you might find your weight loss stalls when you use it. Some people tolerate erythritol (sugar alcohol) just fine and others wind up with diarrhea.

The problem, according to some studies, seems to be that if our brain even senses sweetness, meaning *we taste something sweet*, it initiates an insulin response in our bodies. So even though the sweetener itself technically shouldn't affect us the same as sugar, in reality it does.

Besides releasing insulin, which tells the body to store fat, that sweet taste can also trigger cravings. Once we taste something sweet, we naturally want more of it. To your body, storing fat means you're more likely to survive the hard, cold winter when food is scarce. Even "safe" sweeteners can wind up causing us to overeat, but again, this doesn't happen for everyone.

It's your job to keep track of how much sweetener you're using and notice what's happening with your body. Are your sugar cravings worse? Are you moody and irritable? Is your weight loss stalled? Keeping track and maintaining 100% honesty are the keys to figuring out your body's response to all types of sweeteners.

## MYTH #5: SALT IS DANGEROUS.

"Salt causes dehydration."

"Salt causes high blood pressure."

"Salt causes heart attacks."

"Salt is bad for your kidneys."

These are all statements you've probably heard about salt, and you're probably as terrified of salt as you are of fat. After all, ever since the misguided 1977 government dietary guidelines were passed we've been flooded with warnings about the dangers of salt. Like fat, salt has been unfairly blamed for problems actually caused by sugar.

As we've already established, you cannot lose weight in the presence of insulin because insulin's job is to store fat. A salt deficiency can cause insulin levels to elevate, which means an increased risk of weight gain. That's the opposite of what we want!

A low-salt diet may also promote insulin resistance, one of the tell-tale signs that prediabetes, or even type-2 diabetes, is imminent.

"Cristy, what about people with high blood pressure? Don't they need to stay away from salt?"

There's mounting evidence that low-salt diets increase the likelihood your blood platelets will stick together and clog your arteries, which puts you in *more* danger of a cardiovascular event, not less.

What's more, our bodies cannot produce salt. We lose salt when we sweat, drink caffeine, suffer from untreated sleep apnea, have thyroid issues or if we have gut issues, like leaky gut syndrome, where nutrients from the food we eat aren't properly absorbed.

Another thing you need to know about salt is that on a clean, high-fat diet like the Code Red Lifestyle, we NEED salt. When you follow the Code Red program, you're not eating foods that hang onto sodium. Between that and all the water we drink, our bodies may experience a drop in electrolytes, including sodium.

Eating salty foods (good ones) like pickles and bacon, and salting your food with a good quality sea salt, are simple ways to replenish your sodium. That's right - no more bland, boring food for you with Code Red! Salt your meat, eggs, and veggies, buy salted butter, and enjoy all the flavor salt can bring out in your food.

One more thing. The stark-white table salt you see on supermarket shelves is processed, bleached, and full of chemicals. Use a good quality mineral salt, like Redmond Real Salt. You can also use Himalayan pink salt.

Salt is not your enemy!

## MYTH #6: YOU NEED DAIRY FOR CALCIUM.

Let's talk milk. Did you know humans are the only species that drinks another species' milk? In addition, we are the only species that continues to drink milk after we've been weaned. These are some of the reasons I am not a big fan of milk. I stopped drinking it over a decade ago and except for the heavy cream I put in my coffee, I consume very little dairy. People weren't meant to drink milk throughout their lives, but we were all taught that dairy is a major food group. So many people continue to consume it unnecessarily.

So what's the deal with milk? Most parents give their kids milk. After all, "It does a body good," right? Studies show that one glass of whole milk is nutritionally equal to two glasses of skim, or even 1% or 2% milk. Skim milk has had most or all of the fat removed. What happens when you take all the fat out of something? It tastes awful. If you give kids skim milk, they're just going to ask for chocolate syrup to make it taste better. Give them whole milk if they must have milk.

The fact is, we as a society have been brainwashed over the past 40 years into thinking we need to drink milk. "You need milk to get your calcium." Bull crap. You get more calcium from spinach and chia seeds than you could ever get from milk. Some research indicates that milk actually leaches calcium from your bones, not the other way around. When I need to lose some weight for a photo shoot, the dairy is the first thing to go.

If you must have dairy in your coffee, I really do recommend heavy cream. Even for you folks using half-and-half—the heavy cream is more calorie-dense, but you need so much less of it to cream up your coffee. It has plenty of fat to keep you full and it has far less sugar than half-and-half or milk. Better yet, try some delicious non-dairy milk alternatives, such as unsweetened almond, coconut, cashew, macadamia, or flax milk. Personally, my favorite is flax milk. The consistency is closest to that of cow's milk.

Dairy in general is not going to spike your blood sugar, unless it's ice cream or something with a ton of added sugar. Some dairy foods can be tolerated in weight-loss mode without showing up on the scale. Sour cream, cream cheese, cottage cheese, and heavy cream are all okay if you consume the full-fat variety. Just be very careful to measure and log how much you're eating, so there are no surprises.

Remember that even the full-fat versions of the dairy foods I just mentioned are inflammatory and that alone may prevent you from losing weight. If you find you stall on days you eat dairy, it might be best to cut it out for a while.

But...but...cheese!

As long as we're being honest, let's consider cheese for a minute. It's got no sugar or carbs and it's a great source of fat. So we ought to be able to roll around in a huge tub of Brie with no regrets, right?

Theoretically *yes*, but cheese is extremely calorie-dense. That means there are a *lot* of calories packed into one little ounce of the stuff. (One ounce is roughly 100 grams, for you metric folks.) Different cheeses have different calorie counts, but in general one ounce of hard cheese is 110 calories. There's really no way to know what one ounce actually is unless you slice it and weigh it.

One day I did just that. I sliced it, I weighed it, and I found out that it's not very big at all. You could easily go back for a second, third, fourth, or fifth slice of cheese. Heck, it's easy to polish off half a block without even thinking about it. Pretty soon, you've packed on 500 to 1,000 extra calories and you have no idea why you're gaining weight! And hey, when cheese is melted all ooey-gooey in a spinach dip or on a pizza, who knows exactly how much you're eating? It's really hard to tell.

You've got to track everything. Become a food scientist. Log what you eat, how much, how often—research it. All these years you've been told there's something wrong with you and that's why you can't lose weight. In fact, it could just be the math that's been keeping you fat. Be honest with yourself, that's all I ask.

## MYTH #7: HEALTHY WHOLE GRAINS ARE PART OF A BALANCED DIET.

"Healthy whole grains" have been touted as part of a balanced diet for decades, but things really took off in that arena with, once again, the misguided 1977 government dietary guidelines. We're told we need the nutrients and fiber from "healthy whole grains," and without them, we'll suffer vitamin deficiencies and make ourselves sick.

Here's what we're *not* told...

We currently have a massive wheat industry in the United States. The continent of North America produces enough wheat to feed 11 billion people, even though we're just under 8 billion total human beings on the entire planet. Because we have an overabundance of wheat, the wheat industry has been very proactive in inventing uses for wheat and parts of wheat (like gluten, which we'll talk about later).

Wheat, like sugar, is EVERYWHERE—in both food and non-food products. Our bodies and our society are saturated with it—in far greater quantities than our bodies were designed to handle. That's true whether or not it's whole wheat.

Here's the deal—all grains spike blood sugar, requiring our bodies to produce more insulin. In fact, whole wheat bread can actually spike your blood sugar higher and faster than most candy bars. The word "grains" includes whole wheat, rye, spelt, rice, oats, even corn. Since you cannot lose weight in the presence of insulin, eating a diet rich in "healthy whole grains" is not healthy at all.

Cut out the "healthy whole grains" (and all the other grains as well) and you'll not only lose weight, you'll feel so much better.

## MYTH #8: ALL GLUTEN-FREE FOOD IS HEALTHY.

Gluten is as poorly understood as fat and salt, and it seems like everyone has an opinion about it.

It's been demonized to the point where people think gluten is the root of all their problems, which is just how the food industry likes it. Meanwhile, they're eating copious amounts of sugar and processed foods. Funnily enough, the average person can't even tell you what gluten is, so let's clear that up right now.

Gluten is a naturally occurring protein found in wheat and other grains. Nothing more.

Now is it a problem for some people? Yes, absolutely.

First, there are the people who've been properly diagnosed and know they suffer from celiac disease. They need to avoid gluten entirely. Celiac is a serious autoimmune disease in which gluten severely damages a person's small intestine. Their bodies react badly to it. It is also hereditary, so a person with celiac disease has a 1 in 10 chance of passing it to their kids. Gluten is a very real problem for these folks.

Some people have what's called non-celiac gluten sensitivity, which means their bodies don't make the enzyme to break gluten down. These people also need to be careful around the stuff, because it can attack your body's neural tree. Because your body's neural tree is connected to everything, non-celiac gluten sensitivity can manifest in everything from acne to heartburn to brain disorders that mimic mental illness.

Non-celiac gluten sensitivity is not diagnosable in most hospitals. That means, in order to determine whether you have it, you have to eliminate it from your life for at least a month (though you'll probably notice a difference sooner), then add it back and see what happens.

Gluten is added to all sorts of things including makeup, processed foods, nutritional supplements, beverages, baby formula, pet foods, and a lot of other products. That means ingesting it isn't the only way to be exposed to it. For some people, simply not eating it is enough to help. For others, even external contact with gluten, such as in makeup that touches their skin, can cause side effects.

Remember how I told you that the food industry went crazy slapping low-fat on everything to convince you it's healthy? They're doing the same thing with gluten-free. Look at the processed foods in your local supermarket, and you'll find items labeled "gluten-free" are also packed with sugar and chemicals. Sugar-soaked processed food is sugar-soaked processed food, whether or not it contains gluten or fat.

It would be laughable if it weren't so sad. People spend their hard-earned money on gluten-free breads and crackers believing they are getting healthier, yet nothing changes! That's because it's still bread, folks. It's still crackers. The simple carbohydrates that convert into sugar are all still there. Get rid of the carbs and sugar, get rid of the grains, and you'll feel better.

None of the foods you eat with the Code Red Lifestyle have gluten in them. No grains, no wheat, no gluten. No problem.

Does all this mean you can never eat pizza or a sandwich for the rest of your life? Nope. But in weight-loss mode, you're naturally avoiding gluten because you're avoiding grains in order to avoid stalling your weight loss. When you get down to your goal weight, you may be able to have an occasional slice of pizza or English muffin and be just fine—if your system can handle it. You may find that reintroducing gluten-containing foods causes heartburn, fatigue, headaches, or any other number of unpleasant side effects.

About 20 years ago, I suffered from IBS so badly that I was on medication for it. I was intimately familiar with that fear of eating anything that might trigger those agonizing sharp pains. I was afraid to engage in any activity that might trigger an attack. I couldn't stray too far from a bathroom. It was awful. Once I started eating by the Code Red rules and cut out all grains, sugars, and simple carbs, my IBS was 100% cured. Seriously, when I stopped eating inflammatory foods, the symptoms just disappeared and I stopped taking all that medication.

These days, my body is healthy and there's little or no inflammation.

So I can eat the occasional piece of pizza or sugary treat and not suffer any ill effects. But if I were to disregard the rules regularly, the inflammation would return and I'd suffer those painful episodes all over again. No thanks!

Real, wholesome natural food will not irritate a healthy digestive system. Unfortunately, a healthy digestive system is something few people have in today's world, but following the Code Red program can help you get there.

## MYTH #9: A CALORIE IS A CALORIE.

Calories. Just the word is enough to make some people shiver. Calories have such a negative connotation, but they're highly misunderstood. What exactly is a calorie? There is a long, scientific definition, but basically, it's a unit of energy. It's not evil, it's not bad. It's just energy. You need calories to live. We can't function without a certain number of calories. So why are people so scared of them?

We all know that too many calories can make us fat, but that is only half the story. The typical Western diet is loaded with "empty calories." These are calories with no nutrients. They are manufactured foods that contain plenty of energy, but are also devoid of any wholesome substance. Calories don't make you fat; EMPTY calories make you fat.

You can actually starve yourself while eating loads of processed food, because you're eating calories without nourishing your cells. If your joints ache or your skin is bad, this could be why. You haven't been providing your body with the nutrition it needs to work at optimal performance. Your cells are crying out for nutrition, and YOU'RE HUNGRY ALL THE TIME. Sound familiar?

You keep eating more and more processed junk—maybe even "healthy" processed junk—but your body never gets the nutrition it needs. So many Americans are incredibly sick because of this cycle. They're malnourished and fat at the same time. They're so hungry, even though they consume an enormous amount of food.

It wasn't always like this. Decades ago, we ate fewer calories but enjoyed higher nutrient levels. People from outside the U.S. don't have obesity problems like we do, mainly because their food is higher in nutrients than it is in calories. Before we became a fast-food nation, Americans were like that too. Heart disease, metabolic syndrome, and type II diabetes were not the problems they are now. People ate real food with real nutrients.

We have to get back to eating for nutrition!

Take an avocado, for example. What is it? It's mostly fat. What is fat? Fat is energy, and calories are the units we measure the energy in. Fat actually has the highest energy yield of all the foods you eat. One gram of avocado has twice as much energy stored in it than a gram of grilled chicken breast. When you eat fat, you get more energy bang for your buck.

That's why Code Red Rebels eat fat.

An avocado is higher in calories than a scoop of fat-free ice cream, but it's not the avocado that will make you fat. Here's why...

While there are carbs in an avocado (about 18g), there's also a lot of fiber (about 15g). Fiber helps regulate the effects of the carbohydrate. In this example, you're only *absorbing* about 3g of carbohydrate. Which means the avocado comes in way lower in carbs and sugar than the ice cream. When you're figuring this out for yourself, you can simply subtract the grams of fiber from the grams of carbohydrate to find out how much sugar you're absorbing. This is called finding your "net carbs."

Even more importantly, that avocado has plenty of nutrients that your body needs to function at its best, like vitamin E, vitamin C, folate, and potassium. That fat-free ice cream? It has nothing. It's packed with sugar instead, which your body will store as energy (fat) for later. Worse, you'll still feel hungry even after eating a large serving. An avocado, with all its fat, will nourish your body. The fat-free ice cream will leave your body starved. Avocados, bread, sugar-free ice cream—they all have calories. They're all forms of energy. However, the bread and the ice cream are empty calories. They give your body nothing except sugar to store in your body as fat.

I write carefully balanced nutrition plans for all Code Red custom program clients for this very reason. Most people are used to consuming huge amounts of empty calories every day, including toxic levels of sugar and carbs. The Code Red Lifestyle flips that script. By eliminating the chemically-engineered, manufactured food, you can heal your body by eating calories full of nutritious proteins and fats. You can heal your life with nutrient-rich calories.

## CALORIES IN, CALORIES OUT

There's a huge myth out there that all calories are equal, and that if you simply restrict your calories, you'll lose weight. Here's the deal. A calorie is not a calorie: 1,000 calories of cake is going to be processed completely differently than 1,000 calories of steak. And it will show up on your body completely differently. The cake is full of sugar and not much else. It goes to your liver, spikes your blood sugar, and your body stores those calories as fat. You feel high for a little while, then you crash and want another slice. The steak, on the other hand, has protein, fat, and other nutrients your body needs. There's a slow steady release of energy, with no spikes or crashes.

One more thing—whether you burn a calorie running or sleeping, you've still burned a calorie. So the whole idea that you can just exercise away that piece of cake is a huge fallacy. I mean, in theory you can, but you would have to run for *hours* to burn 1,000 calories. You'll blow out your knee (or your heart) before you ever get rid of that big slice of cake you ate last night.

Just don't eat the cake in the first place, m'kay?

I know that's easier said than done. We'll talk more about how many calories you actually need later in the book. By the end of this book, you'll know how to avoid those sugary empty calories without feeling deprived at all.

## MYTH #10: PRODUCTS LABELED "ALL-NATURAL" ARE HEALTHIER.

How many "all-natural" foods and weight-loss products have you come across? They seem to be endless, don't they? The truth is, food and diet marketing companies are smart. They know that you're more likely to try a product if it's all-natural.

The labeling laws are pretty lax about what has to be in a product in order to use the term "all-natural." If they were to be 100% honest, the label would say "Um, maybe about 8% natural."

The other thing is, just because something is all-natural doesn't necessarily mean it is good for you. Think about it, poison ivy is all-natural. People have died from taking "all-natural" diet products, because they didn't know how the ingredients would interact with their bodies and any other medication or supplement they were taking at the time. This isn't to say that every all-natural product is going to kill you, but don't trust that something is good for you or safe just because of some marketing copy on the label.

As for foods labeled all-natural, they are typically marked up in price with no guarantee they actually are "all-natural." This is especially rampant with foods labeled organic. Ideally, yes, we'd all have access to clean, home-grown produce and meat from animals that are treated humanely. But an "all-natural" food label on a product is no guarantee of any of that, and eating organic is not a necessary step to taking your life back on this program.

Don't trust the marketing companies to have your best interests at heart. Educate yourself, so that if you choose to spend your money on higher-quality foods, higher-quality foods are what you are actually getting.

## MYTH #11: YOU NEED TO TAKE SUPPLEMENTS AND GO ON PERIODIC JUICE CLEANSES TO STAY HEALTHY.

Why is something as important as vitamins and minerals so controversial? Some people say you absolutely need to take supplements and to buy their very expensive brand. Others say you get enough from your food and not to worry about it. My opinion falls somewhere in the middle. When you eat real food, you will be consuming a good portion of the vitamins and minerals you need to survive. But depending on where you live, and where your food comes from, there may be more or less actual nutrition in that head of broccoli.

For one thing, the soil in certain areas has been depleted of its natural ability to supply nutrients to plants. Spinach grown in California will have a completely different nutritional makeup than the same variety grown in Florida. Another consideration is how long that food has been in transit to your store, your fridge, and your plate. If you can go out back, pick your own food from a garden, and cook it within 10 minutes, you're getting the maximum nutrition that soil can provide. If you buy fresh produce in the grocery store, it may have been picked weeks ago. In some cases, frozen produce can actually have *more* nutrition than the fresh stuff simply because it was frozen within hours of being picked. It's so confusing. What do you really need?

First of all, please know your body will cleanse itself. It will heal itself. It can do that. It's amazing!

Now, it only makes sense that if you're trying to "reset" and rid your body of toxins, you can't be adding new ones in at the same time, right? You can't cleanse or detox and still be drinking beer at night, you know what I'm saying? It's counterproductive. Eating a doughnut on the way to work? Not gonna help. Even starting your morning off with Raisin Bran. You're just giving your body extra work to do. Your body can handle itself, as long as you're not creating this perpetual cycle of crap.

It's a good idea to check with your medical professional and maybe even get some bloodwork done, if you think you might be vitamin deficient. Otherwise, as far as the Code Red Lifestyle goes, there are only two supplements I suggest: Vitamin D3 and magnesium, because it's a rare case when someone is not highly deficient in these two.

These are also important because when you eat a high-fat, low-carb diet, your body will flush out the electrolytes you need to keep vital functions going. When you're low on these electrolytes, especially magnesium, it will often show up as muscle cramps. If that happens to you, don't panic. The magnesium will help.

Also, make sure you get a truly high-quality brand. Most of the brands you see in supermarkets and pharmacies are stuffed with inflammatory fillers, have added sugar, and are made from low-grade ingredients (like rocks and horse urine—for real). I learned this after getting my own blood work done. My nurse practitioner said, "I thought you were taking vitamin D?" I explained I was taking 5,000 units every day. Then she said, "Well, it's not even showing up in your bloodwork."

We discovered that I was taking a low-quality brand and was only absorbing about 30% of the dose. So we switched to a high-quality brand, and I now get a 70% absorption rate. So make sure you're using a good-quality supplement. I take my own Code Red brand of D3 and magnesium. A reputable company named Xymogen creates them for me. You can ask your doctor what they recommend. Not all supplement brands are created equal.

Once you've got the garbage out of your system—you've detoxed all the chemicals and sugar and your system is squeaky clean—then what? Are you going to go right back to the doughnuts and coffee? It's no wonder people's systems burn out and become diseased.

Yes, it's worth the work to detox your body. No, you don't need to buy anything to help it. Just eat clean. Drink water. And don't mess it up when you're done. Don't fall for the advertising about detoxing shakes or pills or powders. Your body knows how to take care of itself. It just needs a little bit of help from you, okay?

As for supplementation in general, no amount of supplements, even high-quality ones, will "fix" you if your diet is terrible. You could easily spend thousands of dollars a month on supplements trying to accomplish what can be achieved easily by eating real food, drinking water, and sleeping.

If you insist on taking any supplements, first ask yourself, "Why do I think I need this?" If you don't have a compelling answer, it might be that you don't need that supplement at all.

## MYTH #12: ALCOHOL IS OKAY TO DRINK IN MODERATION.

No alcohol in weight-loss mode. Period.

Even if you don't drink those sweetened fruity umbrella drinks, alcohol metabolizes in the liver and turns into sugar and that's what we're trying to avoid. I've never seen anyone experience consistent weight loss while drinking alcohol. Just don't, okay?

Another issue with alcohol is that it makes you lose your inhibitions. While you might not be worried about dancing on tabletops or drunk-texting your ex, you could seriously damage your weight-loss efforts. You're not going to care about your commitment to yourself and you're much more likely to throw caution to the wind and eat whatever snack foods are put in front of you. Think about it. What else do you do when you're drinking? You eat! Peanuts. Pretzels. Pizza. Buffalo chicken wings. None of these are Code Red-approved.

So just get used to the idea that you're not going to have that vodka for a while. It won't kill you to go without while you're losing weight. If your friends give you a hard time, you can offer to be a designated driver or simply say, "I'm a Rebel."

## DRINKING ALCOHOL IN MAINTENANCE MODE

Once you've lost all your weight, it's okay to start drinking alcohol again, if you want to. Of course, you may feel you did just fine without it and decide you don't really need it. Personally, I just don't think it's worth the calories. So I rarely drink...but it's okay if you do. I want to make you aware of some things, though, because alcohol is a slippery slope back to being overweight.

Let's talk about wine for a minute, shall we? The medical community recommends that a woman should have one glass of wine per day. Men can have two. (I know, it hardly seems fair, right? We birth the babies, and they get to have more wine!) Here's the catch though. Those recommendations are based on a 4 to 5-ounce glass. When I ask a custom program client if they drink any alcohol, a lot of people say yes. Then I ask them how much. They say, "Oh, just one glass." What they mean by "just one glass" is about 12 ounces. Which is actually 3 glasses according to the recommendations.

Go ahead. Pour yourself a "normal" glass of wine, then pour it into a measuring cup and see for yourself. You'll be shocked. It doesn't look like much. Just a typical amount. But it's 3 times more than is recommended. Wine is full of sugar, especially whites and blushes.

Don't get me wrong. I'm not judging how much alcohol you drink. If you choose to drink 3 times the daily limit or a bottle a night, that's your business. You can live your life however you want. Just don't lie to yourself about it. Be honest with yourself and fully understand what and how much you're putting into your body.

I see so many people beating themselves up because they can't lose weight. They blame themselves. They think there's something wrong with them. They even start to hate their bodies. It breaks my heart because there's *nothing* wrong with them. Their bodies are working just fine. The problem is the math. They are consuming 3 times more calories than they think they are.

Yet again, the math is keeping you fat. The math is making you feel crappy. So be honest with yourself. Make sure you truly know how much you are drinking and what that's doing to your weight-loss and maintenance efforts.

## MYTH #13: HIGH CHOLESTEROL MEANS YOU'RE GOING TO DIE.

Sooner or later, the topic of cholesterol comes up for anyone considering a nutrition program like Code Red, where we consume a lot of healthy dietary fat.

Fat has taken the blame for a lot of health problems that are actually caused by sugar, and high cholesterol is another example of this. It's a complicated and misunderstood topic. While I am not a cholesterol scientist, I do want to pass on what I've learned about the latest information on cholesterol, so you can do your research and judge for yourself.

First, let's talk about what cholesterol is. Cholesterol is a white, almost soapy substance that can be found in many places in your body, including your brain. It's a critical part of healthy brain function and normal hormone production. One of the big concerns you've probably heard about cholesterol is that eating foods containing a lot of cholesterol is what raises your cholesterol and that's dangerous.

This is a distorted version of the truth.

Your body actually *makes* cholesterol in response to the foods you eat. It doesn't get cholesterol from the foods themselves.

Another place people get confused is on the issue of good cholesterol and bad cholesterol, which you may have heard called HDL and LDL, respectively.

LDL is the so-called "bad cholesterol," and we've all been taught to demonize it as a risk factor for heart disease and strokes. Blaming LDL cholesterol for heart attacks and strokes is like blaming firemen for responding to the scene of a fire. LDL *responds* to the inflammation in your arteries; it does not cause the inflammation in the first place.

Another thing to be aware of is that LDL is only dangerous in the presence of high blood sugar. Why? High blood sugar causes LDL particles to become sticky and that is when they may cling to your arterial walls and cause blockages. On Code Red, we eliminate foods that cause high blood sugar, which means we're eliminating the foods responsible for sticky LDL particles.

Did you know that most people who suffer heart attacks have what's considered NORMAL cholesterol levels? They also very often have metabolic syndrome, pre-diabetes, or even full-on diabetes.

Once again, sugar is the problem here.

Cholesterol is not the boogeyman we've been led to believe. Do your own research and if at all possible, find a doctor who's up to date on the latest information about cholesterol and high-fat eating.

## MYTH #14: THERE ARE GOOD FOODS AND BAD FOODS

"Why is [insert food here] bad?"

That's a question I get a lot from people new to the Code Red Lifestyle after they get a look at the Foods to Avoid side of the Code Red foods list. Modern humans eat food for every reason they can think of—except actually being hungry. As a result, our emotions get pretty tangled up when it comes to food. Here's a great example of what I mean.

Imagine yourself in a bakery. You're walking the length of the glass case and peering down on all the sugary treats for sale. As you walk the case you're thinking to yourself, with each item, "I'm turning down that one, that one, those ones, that too..." As you walk to the end, you have turned down every treat. At the very end, you think, *Wow, I did such a good job turning down all those treats. I should reward myself with this croissant here at the end. After all, it's not as bad as the German chocolate cake.*

We face our hardest temptations at night, right? That's because we've made good, strong, conscious choices all day. By the time you get home, your willpower is stretched pretty thin. You have worked hard all day, put the kids to bed, and you're relaxing in front of the TV. You were so good all day, so you think it's time for a reward.

Hear me...

Nothing could be more detrimental to your success than rewarding or punishing yourself with food!

It is hard, I know. We were all conditioned as children to view food as a reward. "When you finish your homework, you can have a snack." Or "You got a D in math? Well, no dessert for you for a month, young man!"

Unfortunately, our society has always used food as a reward. We celebrate every occasion with food—both the good and the bad, the weddings and the funerals. That mentality is a big reason we have the hang-ups with food that we do. The inappropriate emotional relationships we have with food all come from using it as a reward, or making it the focal point of a celebration.

Let's talk about comfort food. Macaroni and cheese. It's *chemicals* folks, and nothing more. I know in your mind it's emotionally tied to Grandma, but macaroni and cheese is just a shot of sugar to your system. Is that comfort? No. It's a high. It's a direct deposit to the bank of belly fat. You don't need it. Besides, your Grandma would probably be prouder knowing you were feeling healthy and happy rather than chowing down on food that's bad for your body.

Food isn't comfort.

Food isn't a reward, and it's not a punishment either.

People, food is fuel. That's all it is.

It takes a lot of hard work and brain retraining to make this stick, but food is just fuel. You put it into your body to help it work at peak efficiency. It is detrimental to put things in your stomach that don't belong there. You only have about two ounces of space in your stomach. Picture a shot glass. That is how much space you have; that is all you need to fill.

So if you only have two ounces of space, and your body needs the fuel in that space, you should put the best possible fuel in there, right? Anyone who has raised children knows how little space there is in an infant's bottle. But what goes into that bottle has to be optimal, doesn't it? It has to be clean for that little baby to grow and be healthy.

One of your tasks is to remind yourself, as often as you need to for it to sink in, that food is fuel. You need it. You don't withhold gas from your car and expect it to keep running. You need wholesome, nutritious food to be at your very best. If you have a bad day, if you make a mistake at work, or whatever the case may be, you still feed yourself a good, wholesome meal.

At the same time, you only give your body what it needs. If you're doing really well, reward yourself with a new blouse or a movie ticket, not food. Cramming a bunch of junk into that two-ounce space is only going to hurt you.

I've had clients who wouldn't log any food. They would skip meals entirely as a punishment for not losing any weight the day before. That is not okay, either. You can't operate at your best if you're not giving your body what it needs. That is punishing yourself with food and not only is it wrong, it doesn't work. You can't just stop feeding yourself.

No matter how big you are, no matter how old you are, it is never too late to change your relationship with food. It's certainly not too late for your kids, if you have them. *You are in charge of you* and you have a responsibility to feed yourself wholesome, real food every single day. It is the fuel your body needs.

Food is not "good" or "bad." There's food that nourishes you and food that doesn't. Labeling "good food" and "bad food" is just another way to pile on emotional baggage like guilt and shame when it comes to food.

"But Cristy, what about all the 'avoid' foods on the Code Red food list? Aren't they bad?" No. They are there because I know for a fact they stall or prevent weight loss. Nothing else.

Food is fuel. It's not good or bad, just like it's not a reward or a punishment.

## MYTH #15: HUNGER IS BAD.

When people talk about diets, one of the first things out of their mouths is "But, but, I don't want to feel *hungry!*" Fear of hunger has really gotten completely out of hand in today's world. To be clear, I'm not talking about families who are truly destitute and aren't sure when they might have their next meal. Nor am I talking about people who claim they're "always hungry" (which, by the way, only happens because they eat a boring, low-fat diet with foods that either have very little nutrition, or that spike insulin.)

I'm talking about normal hunger. The kind that's supposed to happen. The kind that's the body's normal response to needing more fuel. The kind that happens naturally as a result of eating real food, drinking water, and sleeping well. (Yes, lack of sleep also leads to hunger.)

We eat so much food in today's society that we're used to feeling stuffed all the time. So much so that the actual sensation of hunger is alien and scary to a lot of people. I've had clients start the Code Red Lifestyle feeling absolutely terrified of experiencing hunger, as if a couple hours of the hunger sensation meant they were going to drop dead on the spot. True hunger is nothing more than a chemical signal from your brain telling you it could use some more fuel.

As I tell my clients on a daily basis, "Ain't nobody gonna die from skipping a meal and ain't nobody gonna die from feeling the sensation of hunger."

That doesn't mean I expect you to feel ravenous 24/7 either. Fortunately, when you eat the rich, delicious, full-fat foods we eat on Code Red, drink your water, and get your sleep, that won't happen. Client after client, success story after success story—they all tell me how shocked they were by the fact that they were rarely hungry.

Stop letting the sensation of hunger frighten you into staying overweight and sick. Hunger, when it takes place on a healthy lifestyle like Code Red, is a GOOD thing. It means your body's working the way it's supposed to.

## MYTH #16: MAINTAINING A HEALTHY WEIGHT IS IMPOSSIBLE FOR ME BECAUSE _____.

If I had a nickel for every time someone told me they couldn't lose weight or keep it off because of age, genetics, gender, or having kids, I could retire! At the same time, I get it. Everywhere we turn, we're told things like...

"You'll never get back to your high school weight."

"Weight gain is just a part of getting older."

"You'll gain 15 pounds with every baby."

"It's just how you're built."

Guess what? I have thousands of people who've done my program who have proven every single one of those statements wrong. My friend Cassie is smaller now than she was in high school. That's after having four children.

It's the same with my sister, Cari. Obesity runs in our family, yet we've been able to lose our weight and keep it off by following the Code Red Lifestyle. So have thousands of others, including people who've been heavy since they were kids.

People come in all shapes and sizes. Genetics may influence *some* things, but they are not the be-all, end-all for your size. So what is the be-all, end-all?

Eat real food. Drink water. Sleep.

That prescription works for people who've had kids, for people in their 70s and 80s, for people who've been heavy for as long as they can remember and for people with a family history of obesity.

Myths can be powerful, especially when you've been hearing them all your life. I'm not asking you to magically stop believing whatever you believe. All I'm asking is that you go all-in with the Code Red Lifestyle. See for yourself what can happen when you follow the Code Red rules, eat the approved foods, and follow the "avoid foods" list while in weight loss mode.

You absolutely CAN maintain a healthy weight as a part of a happy, healthy lifestyle.

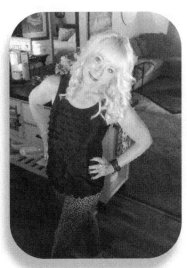

I've never been really overweight and there have been times when I've been really skinny. But right after we had grandkids, I noticed I was feeling a bit squishy around the middle. At the time, I thought, *that's okay, I'm going to be one of those soft, huggable grandmas.* What I was really doing was convincing myself that I wanted to be soft and squishy. My grandmothers were like that and I figured that's how it would be for me. I just thought getting larger was what happened when you got to be in your 50s and had grandkids.

Even though I was trying to accept this whole "squishy grandma" thing, deep down I really didn't want to. The extra weight bugged me. About that time, my daughter Cristy came home to visit us. This was when she was a personal trainer in New York and hadn't yet developed the Code Red nutritional lifestyle, so she had me running up mountains and doing all this exercise to get the weight off.

Now I don't mind being active. I'll go for a walk or ride a horse, but I don't really like to exercise and all this work wasn't exactly melting the pounds off. So I started thinking about creative ways to hide those few extra pounds, like changing my hairstyle or my clothes.

Sometime later, Cristy really figured out the nutrition component and started helping people experience some amazing weight loss. I started watching her videos and we talked on the phone. I began to really look at what I was cooking and eating.

I figured I could do anything for 30 days, so I had her write up a nutrition plan for me. Back then, I was in pain all the time, especially in my fingers and wrists. I just figured I was getting older and this must be arthritis. That happens when you get older, right? I wasn't on any medication or anything, but the pain was there every night. It didn't really go away until I went to sleep.

So I followed the plan she made for me. I didn't cheat at all. The first week was tough—especially getting off sugar—but other than that it was pretty simple. I lost the weight I wanted to and felt great. I was so busy that I just went about my life as normal.

**Then about a month into it, I stopped dead in my tracks one day. I looked at my hands and realized the pain was gone. It wasn't just a little bit better—it was 100% gone!**

I told Cristy about it and she said, "Mom, I think it's the grains. You've gotten rid of the inflammation." That made sense. I didn't really think any more about it, until I got a craving for some Chinese food. I went out and picked up some takeout chicken with rice. Oh, the next morning...I was puffy, my knuckles hurt—it was terrible, and that's when I got it. Everything my daughter had said about the grains was right.

At that point, I had two choices. I could moan and groan, suffer through the pain, take my pain relievers and just chalk it up to old age. Or I could knock that crap off and stop eating the foods that made me hurt! Instead I could choose to eat the food that made me wake up with a burst of energy so I could do the housework, cook the meals and be out the door to work by 8 a.m. After I realized that, I really had no choice but to follow the Code Red rules.

I was excited about the 20-pound weight loss, but I was so much more excited to be pain-free. These days, whenever I eat pasta or accidentally have some grains in a sauce or something, I pay for it the next morning. The pain comes back every time.

I know my numbers. I know the rules. Sometimes I still let my weight creep up or I get behind on my water, but once it gets to a certain point, I have to just say, "No more." That's when I have to get serious about following the rules for weight-loss mode until I get back to where I want to be.

My husband, Larry, was able to stop taking so many medications after he started the Code Red Lifestyle. He loves to go hunting and be outdoors. Now he can run around with the grandkids and then go chop a tree down. We aren't just "being" grandparents. We are "doing" the grandparent thing. We're active. We're running around and swimming and playing games outside. We are actively participating in their lives and that's how it should be.

Here's how I see it: If you do nothing, in a month or a year you'll be exactly where you are now or worse. If you take action, follow the rules and make friends with the other Code Red Rebels, you're going to feel better. I want to be as healthy as I can for as long as I can. I've seen so many people take their lives back with Cristy's program, I know that anyone can do this. Age is not an excuse.

**Don't for one second believe that lie that you're "too old" to lose weight and turn your life around.** Whatever age you are, it doesn't matter. You can absolutely get healthier and feel better when you eat the right foods, drink water, and get enough sleep.

## 3-YEAR UPDATE

Quite a lot has changed, namely that I got divorced after 48 years of marriage. I also sold my favorite house ever and relocated to Boise.

My life this past year and a half has been one huge uphill struggle. I often think about things like, "How will I make it on my own? What happens if the roof leaks, if the car breaks down, or the water lines freeze? What do I do when I have to get my snow tires on or off?" And some of those things did happen, but guess what? I dealt with it. I did all I could by myself and got help and advice from others when I needed to.

I have never lived alone in all my life, so it was all a bit scary. One thing that really helped was talking with myself a lot, as in problem solving and figuring out the best way to handle something. Then putting on my big girl pants and just doing the hard things. I have actually surprised myself at how efficient and strong I am.

I absolutely KNEW I did not want to add weight gain to my long list of stressors, especially since I've lost another 20 pounds since the first book! That would have been the worst thing I could have done. To make sure it didn't, I stayed in daily contact with my girls for support.

Plus, I never let myself stay down or depressed for more than a day. I do a lot of self-talk and stay vigilant with regard to the thoughts I let in.

The battle for anything is won in the mind, so we need to choose every day to make good choices.

For me, that means absolutely no non-Code Red approved items lurking anywhere in my house. If I'm at the store and pick up something questionable on a whim or during a weak moment, I'll make myself turn it over and read the carb and sugar content. That's usually enough for me to toss it back like a hot potato.

I also need to be held accountable to someone who will ultimately steer me to choose wisely. Making a pact, agreement or challenge with people to whom I'm accountable is a fun and effective way to stay the course.

Don't become complacent in your day-to-day life and don't believe the lies your brain wants to tell you. You WILL be successful. Be positive and keep moving in the right direction. Be present in your life because TODAY is all we really have.

# CHAPTER 10

# REBEL FOR LIFE

NOW THAT YOU understand how to lose the weight, and the simple strategy for keeping it off, it's time to talk about the one thing that can make or break how successful you are on this new path:

Mantras For Life

This entire section is devoted to proven mindsets to succeed both in weight loss mode, and moving forward with the rest of your healthy, happy life. What you're going to learn in this section are things "diet books" will NEVER tell you.

As we've already established, being a Code Red Rebel For Life isn't about diets. It isn't even about weight loss. It's about living a full, healthy, happy life. Sound good? Then let's dive in!

## TRAIN LIKE YOU FIGHT, FIGHT LIKE YOU TRAIN

When I got started in boxing, I learned a very powerful training mantra: We train like we fight and fight like we train.

That means you want fighting in the boxing ring to be no different than fighting during training. Bright lights and people yelling and screaming, like you'd get on fight day, were simulated during training. Even the order I put on and laced up my boots was the same. The more training and "real fights" had in common, the less jarring it was for me on fight day.

I stayed relaxed. I didn't have to think during my fight, because muscle memory and primal instinct took over.

You need to do the same thing. When you create habits for yourself and make choices that'll get you where you want to be, you are in "training." That way, when your "fight day" comes—in the form of stress at work, a fight with your spouse, an unexpected bill, or the kids acting up—you don't have to think about what to do. You've already programmed yourself to react in a way that'll keep you on track.

See, everybody thinks they've got it figured out - until they get "hit." You'll think to yourself, "Oh, I'll just go to that party and figure it out once I get there." Then you show up and find out they are serving chocolate cheesecake, your favorite. You decide just one bite won't hurt. Problem is, it's never just one bite. Next thing you know, you're halfway through your second piece and dreading what the scale's going to say the next morning.

Without the right training, you will get hit, and staying on track will go right out the window. So how do you stop that from happening? Make a plan and stick to it.

Before you go to that gathering where there's gonna be tempting food, before you bake cupcakes for your kid's birthday party, before your next vacation - make a plan to stay on track, and follow that plan. That way, when push comes to shove, you don't "get hit." Instead, you stay on track... and do so without having to depend on *willpower*.

Train like you fight and fight like you train. The more you train yourself to succeed, by making the right choices for yourself, the more successful you'll be on *fight days* like the office holiday party. Getting your mind on board with your new way of life is a sure way to stay on your new path of hope and healing.

Here are my favorite ways to train your brain for success.

## RECOGNIZE MENTAL BLOCKS AT CERTAIN WEIGHTS

Losing weight is a very emotional experience for most people. That's because having a weight problem is not about having a weight problem. It's a symptom of a deeper issue. What that issue is depends on you and your life experience.

Unworthiness is a BIG reason for weight problems. A lot of people subconsciously believe they're unworthy of the effort it takes to lose the weight and live a healthy, happy life. I've had clients who've overeaten themselves into a weight problem in order to punish themselves because they hated themselves so much.

Physical and mental abuse are also very common reasons for a weight problem. People who've been victimized often gain a lot of weight because they believe it'll protect them from being victimized again. It won't, because being victimized isn't about you. It's about the person who hurt you.

Only you can say for sure what that deeper issue might be. If you're losing weight just fine, and suddenly start sabotaging yourself at a certain weight, that deeper issue could be a reason behind the sabotage. I've had clients who weighed 275 pounds make it all the way to 200 pounds, then start sabotaging themselves. Why? Because they hadn't been below 200 in so long, the idea of being in the 100s freaked them out.

I've also had clients self-sabotage because something traumatic happened to them at a certain weight. Maybe they got divorced, or were abused, or someone they cared about passed away. If this sounds a little unbelievable to you, I get it, but I've seen it in my clients enough to know it's a true concern for some people. Mental blocks like this can even hit as you reach goal weight. The idea of being done losing weight is so unbelievable, you self-sabotage and stay 5 or 10 pounds above goal, then wonder "What's wrong with me?!"

There's nothing wrong with you. Stop asking that question.

If you find yourself self-sabotaging at certain weights, here's what you can do:

- Remember that the past is the past. Returning to the weight you were back then is not going to change the past, or make it the present. The empowerment you feel when you move beyond this mental block weight is better than just about anything you can imagine. I'm not invalidating what might have happened to you. I'm pointing out that just because it happened then doesn't mean it's going to happen again just because of a number on the scale.
- If you've never weighed lower than a mental block weight, or it's just been a long time, I understand it's uncharted territory for you. But not allowing yourself to move beyond it and step into that un-

charted territory is not going to help you heal. It's not going to empower you to take your life back. All it will do is to continue to hold you back. Take things a day at a time, and reach out for support.

## MANAGE YOUR EMOTIONAL EATING

For the longest time, I didn't realize I was an emotional eater. Seriously, no clue. Living in New York City was one of the loneliest, most stressful times of my life. Every night, on the way home from working with my personal training clients, I'd buy a one-pound bag of peanut M&Ms. After I got home, I'd watch TV and eat the whole bag in one sitting. Afterwards, I felt sick, and my stomach was distended and uncomfortable. I was in pain, but I was also distracted from my loneliness.

There are so many reasons we emotionally eat. We eat to numb feelings we don't like, we eat to cope, we eat to deal with stress, we eat to punish ourselves, we eat to celebrate and to bond with others. When you eat to feel better, the fact you feel better isn't your imagination. It's biology. Digestion requires two-thirds of your body's energy and that energy has to come from someplace, so your body will pull resources and devote them to digestion. That means it has fewer resources to spare on your emotions.

Think about it. If you're used to coping with emotions like stress, anger, anxiety, or depression, by eating, does the thought of not eating when you feel that way freak you out a little?

If so, you're an emotional eater.

It's nothing to be ashamed of. Most people are, including me. In New York, I got past the peanut M&Ms problem by getting a little help and taking a different route home from work. That way I wasn't passing right by the place where I'd bought the M&Ms so many times.

These days there are still things that trigger me to want to eat emotionally. I remember a time when my husband found me sitting at my desk with a giant tub of almonds between my legs, eating them by the handful. "Cristy, what are you doing?" he asked me, lifting the tub of almonds away.

I was stunned, because I didn't even remember grabbing the almonds, much less eating half of them.

Now that I understand I'm an emotional eater, I have a plan in place to outsmart myself, so that I cope without turning to food. I might contact my mom or sister. I'll go for a run with Annabelle (my dog) to get out of the house and away from the food. I'll even just sit with the emotion for a few minutes and allow myself to feel it, instead of trying to numb it with food. Doing that gets intense sometimes, but afterwards I feel better.

Having an emotional eating problem doesn't mean it has to control you. Awareness of your triggers and a simple plan to outsmart them are the keys. There's no such thing as suppressing your emotions. You might be able to stuff them down with food (or some other numbing behavior) in the moment, but one way or another, they're going to express themselves, and it'll probably be in a way that tears you, or someone you love, down.

Eating your feelings doesn't work. It's a lot healthier to express your feelings, so you can release them and move on. How you express them is up to you. You can take a few minutes of alone time and allow yourself to feel them (without judging yourself for having them), you can write them in a journal, you can call a supportive friend, or pick something from your list of 100 things that make you happy.

## YOU ARE NOT THE PROBLEM; THE PROBLEM IS THE PROBLEM

One of my past clients kept bouncing between success and regression. She would do awesome and lose 30 pounds, but then binge on her husband's junk food. Her husband, at that time, refused to eat healthy and kept his junk food in the house where it didn't belong. My client, who worked so hard to avoid the temptation of unhealthy food in her space every day, eventually broke down.

She would ask, "What's wrong with me?" She told me the junk food didn't even taste good, but she shoved it down anyway. I asked her what she would do if the food wasn't in the cupboard. She said that if it wasn't in the house, she wouldn't eat it. Ding ding ding—we have a winner!

We talked about her options. She was 50% owner of that house, and 50% of that marriage. We talked about asking her husband to keep his junk food somewhere other than the cupboard. Whether it was in his man-cave, his office, the garage, wherever—if it was not in the space she used, then she wouldn't eat it.

We identified her problem, then we solved it. That's what I mean when

I tell you that you are not the problem, the problem is the problem, so just work the problem.

Instead of asking, "What's wrong with me?" or "Why am I so messed up?" focus on identifying the problem. For this client, it was simply a matter of moving her husband's junk food to a bin in a part of the house where she wouldn't have to look at it every day. She already knew she could lose the weight, she just needed the garbage out of her space.

Another past client was a high-powered 1% earner. She led work conferences where she taught people how to do their jobs. After these conferences, she would binge. Again, her response was, "Why do I do this? What's wrong with me?"

My answer: Who cares about why? I don't care about why. I care about how to solve that problem. With this client, I learned that when she got home from a conference, she was alone in the house and headed for the pantry. That's where we found the answer. She went home. She didn't go to the store, she didn't order out. She went to her space and raided her own cupboard.

There were two issues here. On one hand, she had food in her house that she shouldn't have. (One of my three big rules is to keep unhealthy food out of your house and this is why.) The other issue was that when she came out of one of those big conferences, she was running on high energy. She found she needed to go to a hotel or decompress somewhere that wasn't home. Then she could return home and make rational choices about a healthy dinner.

It is up to you to fix your problems. If you want to see a counselor or a therapist to figure out why you have a problem, that's fine. I support that. However you can choose to simply identify and fix the problem.

Do us both a favor and don't put all the stress, blame, and shame on your shoulders. No "What's wrong with me?" No "Why can't I change?" None of that. That is not going to help you push forward. You are not the problem; the problem is the problem. The sooner you can identify the problem, the sooner you can fix it and move forward.

## CONQUER COMPLACENCY

One of the most embarrassing losses in my boxing career happened

CRISTY "CODE RED" NICKEL

during my prime. I had a world title under my belt and was the number two ranked boxer in the world. My next opponent was a no-name fighter from a small town, just like I was when I started. Boy was I sure of myself when I learned who I was up against. I just "knew" I was going to whip her butt.

Instead, I got my butt handed to me.

Why? Because I got complacent. I told myself "I got this," but the reality was, I underestimated her, which is the absolute worst thing you can do when facing an opponent.

Complacency has no place in your healthy new lifestyle. Your brain is wired to seek comfort. It means well, but it doesn't always understand what's best for you in the moment vs. what's best for you long-term. Just like the worst thing you can do in the ring is underestimate your opponent, the worst thing you can do in your healthy new lifestyle is underestimate your brain's yearning for comfort and convenience over what's actually healthy.

This doesn't mean I want you to live in fear or to doubt yourself. The choice to stay with your new lifestyle is a daily recommitment. Complacency has probably gotten the better of you before. We can be really good at talking ourselves out of doing what we know is good for us. Be mindful of this fact and be mindful of your decisions. There are Rebels who've been successful for years (and counting). One reason why is that they get good at identifying complacency and putting a stop to it. You can, too!

## JUST GO LEFT

One cheat sets you back a week. It's true. Here's how I know. In the very early days of Code Red, I allowed my clients to have a cheat meal, where they could eat anything they wanted. Most of them followed their program all week long and lost weight. Then came cheat meal day. They'd gorge on their cheat foods and just like that, gain back all the weight they'd spent a week losing. Finally, I removed cheat meals from weight loss mode entirely, because it dragged that process out for weeks, even MONTHS. When I removed cheat meals, people lost weight a lot faster and were also able to break free from sugar addiction, since they were no longer reintroducing those sugary foods they were addicted to.

Then I noticed a different pattern emerging. Most people stayed on track and got their weight off, but sometimes I'd see clients slip up and then decide, "Well, I already messed up, may as well make it a whole week of slip-ups!"

One slip-up does not need to become a week or even a day of slip-ups. If you have a weak moment, or absent-mindedly lick the beaters while making cupcakes for your kid's birthday party—just go left.

Here's what that means.

My sister, Cari, was driving her youngest daughter to school one day. After dropping her off, Cari had another errand to run, but she wasn't sure how to get there. She asked one of the other moms for directions. The other mom told her to drive straight for a short time, then "just go left."

Not go right, not drive around the block and end up right back where she started.

Just go left.

That's what I want you to do if you slip up. Don't beat yourself up. Don't use it as an excuse to go crazy and flush all your efforts down the toilet. Just go left. Wipe the slate clean and start right back up. One slip-up bite doesn't need to turn into one slip-up meal. One slip-up meal doesn't need to turn into one slip-up day.

None of this is an excuse to play fast and loose with the Code Red program. Do it or don't do it.

If you decide you're doing it and you slip up, forgive yourself. Then just go left.

## PICK YOUR HARD

No matter how skilled you might be at playing soccer, there are times when it's challenging. No matter how beautifully you may play the piano, you put in long, difficult hours to learn. No matter how much you love your children, parenting is hard. Everything in life has moments when it's hard, sometimes a lot of moments in a row. Really, if life were always easy, it wouldn't mean much, would it?

I don't think anyone would argue with me that being obese is hard. You don't have to be on *The Biggest Loser* or *My 600-Pound Life* to be obese. If 30% of your body weight is fat, then you are obese. That means you don't have to weigh 300, 400, or 500 pounds to be in this category. If you weigh 250 pounds and 75 pounds of that is fat, you are obese.

Obesity is hard. Sure you get to eat whatever you want, but your clothes don't fit. You feel like you're going to pass out after climbing a flight of stairs. You don't have the energy to run around in the backyard with your children or grandchildren. Your knees and back ache all the time. Or maybe you have no confidence because you hate the way you look. Or you don't like having sex with your spouse because you don't want to take your clothes off. Obesity is a rough place to be and that is why everyone wants out.

On the flip side, weight loss and real nutrition can be tough too. My clients tell me that my program is hard. Being obese is hard, losing weight is hard and maintaining a goal weight is hard too.

You have to PICK YOUR HARD.

You can choose to be obese and stay in that abusive relationship with food, or you can transform your life with dedication and nutritious food. It's entirely up to you. Don't fool yourself—both options are hard, at least some of the time.

Any way you slice it, you will have to work at something. So my advice to you is to choose the hard that leads to a healthier, happier life for yourself. Just make up your mind that you're going to do it and tackle it head on.

All change is hard, but this change, the commitment you make to improve your life and heal your body, it's a good change. It's the best change... and it's going to make the rest of your life so much easier.

Is it hard? Yes.

Can you do it? Absolutely!

## MAINTAIN FAITH IN THE MIDDLE

You've probably had a lot of moments in your life where the excitement of *the new thing* you're doing has worn off, but the outcome you're after still seems far away. How do you keep going in that middle stretch? How do you just do the grind so you can get where you want to be, instead of falling away again?

The answer is having faith in the middle.

It's grinding on, even when you don't feel like it, even when it's not exciting anymore and even when your outcome still seems a million miles away.

You may have heard the saying, "It's not how you start, it's how you finish." I say it's not how you start OR end. It's what you do in the middle that makes all the difference. The middle is where the rubber meets the road. It's where you either dig in and have faith, or it's where you fizzle out and give up. It's where complacency tries to sneak back in and tell you things like...

"You've already lost so much weight. You've done enough."

"Another friend just told you how good you look. You probably don't need to lose any more weight after all."

"You've done SO well on the program! One little treat won't hurt anything."

Sound familiar?

The middle is where your commitment to your goal will be tested. It is NOT the time to listen to the voice of complacency. It's the time to buckle down, reach out for support and recommit. It's the time to remember that little decisions add up. You didn't end up in this mess overnight. It wasn't one bite of brownie that got you here. It took years of little decisions, stacked one on top of the other.

The great news is that the way out is the same - little decisions - except now you get to make DIFFERENT little decisions that move you into your amazing, healthy new life. The only way those decisions will work is if you keep making them, even if you don't feel like it. As the saying goes, commitment doesn't care how you feel. You do the work because it's taking you where you want to go, regardless of whether your complacency voice would rather sneak in a bag of Cheetos and a diet soda.

There's no avoiding the middle. Diet industry quick fixes want you to believe there is and they count on your belief to sell you more shakes and pills and mail-order frankenfood. Don't fall for it. Face the middle and have faith in me, this program and yourself, to get to the next step on your new path. Stay connected to the real, raw reasons you're doing this. Stay connected to people who support you on this new path. Lean on them if you need help with faith in the middle.

## CONTROL WHAT YOU CAN CONTROL

The feeling of being in control is great, isn't it? It's reassuring. It feels safe. Our brains like it, too, which is one reason it's so jarring when things happen that are outside our control. No matter how good you get at curating what you see in your news feed, or surrounding yourself with like-minded people, or keeping the junk food out of your house, life will throw curveballs your way.

If someone you love passes away unexpectedly, if a natural disaster hits, if a world-changing event pops up seemingly out of the blue and forever impacts our day to day lives—that loss of certainty and control can throw you for a loop.

Our brains hate the unexpected as much as they love the feeling of being in control. Anything that triggers a feeling of no control can really rattle you and...if you allow it to... lead you to do things you wouldn't do otherwise. Escapist behaviors are a common go-to when you feel like you can't control what's happening. Numbing yourself with food, alcohol, drugs, or streaming TV feels more bearable than living with the sensation of no control.

We all have to figure out how to cope, but there are positive ways to cope and not so positive ways to cope. A simple way to tell the difference is to think about the future. When the thing you can't control has passed, will you be better off than you are now, or worse off?

A while back, one of my clients lost her mother. I asked her what she wanted to do and she told me she wanted to continue with her program. "It's the one thing I can control," she told me.

When life feels out of control, controlling what you CAN is how you stay sane. What you put in your mouth (or don't put in your mouth) is something you can control. A lot of people make the choice to put crap in their mouth, but that isn't the way it has to be.

If someone you love dies while you're in weight loss mode and you're tempted to cope by eating yourself out of house and home, ask yourself: When my grief has backed off a little, do I want to weigh less than I do now, or more? Do I want to feel proud of myself for making good choices, or feel like a failure for letting things slip? Which outcome feels better to you?

When life feels out of control, focus on what you CAN control. Namely, *yourself*. You have a say in what you think, feel, and do. Make GOOD choices for yourself. Focus on you and YOUR actions. And reach out for help if you need to.

Luis Aguilar Jr.
Boise, Idaho
Age 33
Lost 140 pounds

I've been overweight since I was a child. By second or third grade, I was already obese. By high school, I had back pain so bad that it affected my ability to sleep. I've been packing on extra weight my entire life.

I knew my eating habits weren't the best. Being single, I always just did what was easiest. I ate out almost every meal, McDonald's or whatever, usually washed down with some Pepsi. It wasn't even satisfying. I snacked between every meal—I was ALWAYS hungry.

If I didn't eat, I'd get headaches and feel shaky. The guys at work knew. They'd be like "Dude, just stop and go eat. You're getting angry." So I'd go get something quick, which was usually more junk. In a few hours, it would all start over again. I hated that feeling, but I felt like there was nothing I could do about it.

I was a cereal addict. That was my thing. I even ate it before bed. I ate pizza, probably four times a week. When I think about all the money I spent on pizza (which is basically poison), it makes me sick.

I thought Subway was a healthier option, so when I was trying to be healthier, I was eating 12-inch subs. But that didn't help me lose weight, and it cost me a lot of money too. No joke, I spent $600 or $700 a month on unsatisfying food that kept me overweight and feeling bad about myself.

Most people saw me as an easy-going, happy-go-lucky guy, but I didn't feel that way. I was depressed. I didn't feel good about myself at all, so I would eat to feel better. Inside, I was always very self-conscious. I always wore big, baggy clothes and sweatpants to hide my size.

I heard about Code Red from my mom. I noticed how healthy she looked and how much more energy she seemed to have. Once when I was over for a visit, she made me a Bulletproof coffee—you know, with butter and heavy whipping cream in it. I was surprised how good it was.

Not long after that, my mom joined one of Cristy's challenges and she really took off with it. That got my little sister Camille interested and she joined the next month's challenge. I thought that was funny, because we always thought of Camille as the skinny one—she was never as big as the rest of us. Every time I came to visit, the two of them were lighter and happier.

When Camille's husband Josh started looking better too, I was like, "Okay guys, what's going on?"

My mom told me about Code Red. "Just read the book and follow the food list."

When I saw the list of foods, I kind of freaked out. My family didn't push it.

Months later, I was getting ready to move and my parents and sister came down to help me. I'm not going to lie—they kicked my ass. I couldn't get up and down the stairs like they did. I was cramping up, out of energy... and my 50-plus-year-old parents were just cruising right along.

So I finally decided to give *The Code Red Revolution* a real read. I don't read much—a book has to really captivate me for me to finish it. I read that book *twice in one night*. I saw myself in those pages. It motivated me. I was really able to relate to Cristy.

I decided to give it my all. I didn't do a custom program—I literally just read the book. The next challenge wasn't until several months later and I didn't want to wait. I marched my happy ass to the pantry and piled up everything I had just bought so I could get rid of it.

I gave some to my roommate and donated the rest to food banks here in Boise. Then I went shopping again—this time with the Code Red list.

Right away, I noticed changes. The detox was pretty hard. My mom and sister had tried to prep me for it, warning that it could take 8 to 10 days. Mine lasted for 18.

I had a lot of stuff to give up though. I was chewing tobacco, drinking at least four Pepsis a day and eating out almost every meal. I was detoxing from YEARS of that. At first, I thought it was going to kill me. I wanted to give up. I called my sister crying, wanting to quit. She told me to hang on and promised me I'd break through.

Sure enough, the very next day, I woke up and felt like a new person. My brain fog had lifted, my energy was up, I just felt great. By that point, 18 days in, I had lost 15 pounds. Since then, I've never looked back.

I still struggle sometimes, still get tempted by the old foods I used to eat, but I know they're no good for me. Even when I broke down and took a bite of something that wasn't on the list, it didn't taste good. My body just didn't want it anymore.

That's what's great about this lifestyle—if you do have a bad day and mess up, you can just start over right away. You don't have to quit just because you screwed up. You know exactly what to do to get back on track. I feel like that's why other diets always failed. If I made one mistake, it was over and I just gave up. With Code Red, my mentality has really changed.

**At first it was a weight-loss journey for me, but once I saw how easy it was to lose the weight, it became more of an everything journey for me.**

I handle stress better than I used to. In fact, my anxiety has gone away. There's so much more to this lifestyle than just weight loss. My whole life transformed and I want other people to know that their lives can too.

My entire family is on Code Red—cousins, aunts, even grandparents. Seeing all that positive change in my family, I know it's real. That's why I stand behind it.

One thing I tell everybody is to watch the NSVs—non-scale victories. At first, you're going to be all about seeing that scale go down. But the NSVs are all the things that make your life better.

Some of mine were really big. My back pain? GONE. I can finally sleep through the night without having spasms. I don't have to pop ibuprofen like Skittles anymore. I even got to jump on a trampoline!

My psoriasis is gone. Years ago, a specialist told me that topical creams weren't going to fix it, that I needed to find another way. Code Red was the solution.

I used to wear size 46 pants—now I'm down to a 29. I'll be able to fly on a plane without the extended belt for the first time in my life. My shirts used to be XXX, but now I wear a medium. I lost five inches around my neck! My shoes have more room in them, my rings and even my hats and sunglasses are too big now.

NSVs are the best, and they're different for everyone. I remember how exciting it was to see my kneecaps for the first time in a long while. That's something most people would take for granted, but it was a victory for me. I have more confidence around my customers, and my performance at work has improved. Seeing all these positive changes in my body proved for me that food is medicine and medicine is food.

When you look for those NSVs, you begin to see them everywhere, including in other people on their own journeys. I see how confident my sisters are. That's the greatest feeling—being proud of the people around you and knowing they're proud of you too. When you're around like-minded people, you support each other.

Even my company's owner told me he was proud of me—that meant a lot. It made me realize that people were watching me and I had a chance to help others change their lives. I'm humbled to have this opportunity. I'm so grateful to Cristy for showing us the way.

At this point, I've lost 125 pounds. I started at 288, and I'm down to 162. When I reached my initial goal weight of 167, I thought that was a real stretch, but I'm still losing. Now I'm focusing on my body fat percentage, but I know it's going to just fall off.

I can resist the food I need to avoid. I can avoid the donuts in the breakroom because for me they're poison. I care more about what I'll be able to enjoy. I'm looking forward to having the BEST summer. I've always liked warm weather, but now I can enjoy it without overheating. I'm excited to take my shirt off and get a tan—something most people take for granted.

For anyone who's overweight and wants to change, sign up for a challenge. It's a game-changer. The support you'll find with that community is so worth it. They're my friends now. We share stories and keep each other going.

The biggest thing I love is Cristy's no-negativity rule, which allows people to be truly vulnerable. Otherwise, I never would have shared my "before" pictures on a public platform. I knew people wouldn't make fun of them or judge me. And they helped inspire other people in the CR community. The first time someone in the group told me I inspired them, it was humbling and it kept me motivated.

This lifestyle is awesome. There's no downside…except maybe a few extra pee breaks on road trips (ha ha). Men, women, kids and old folks—anyone can do this. My 12-year-old nephew even lost weight doing Code Red! Sometimes guys feel like they have to exercise to lose weight. It's the macho way, you know? But you don't have to exercise to lose weight with Code Red. I achieved all my success without breaking a sweat.

If I could tell everyone in the world, I would. Losing weight with Code Red is the easiest hard thing I've ever done. Changing your lifestyle is hard, but living overweight and feeling bad all the time is harder. You have to want it and you have to follow the rules. That's it. It's that simple. Trust Cristy's rules, stick to the food list and give it 30 days.

Don't you owe it to yourself to try?

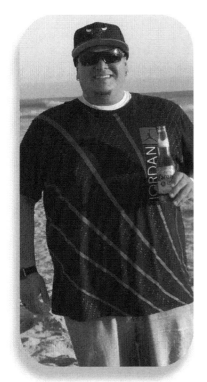
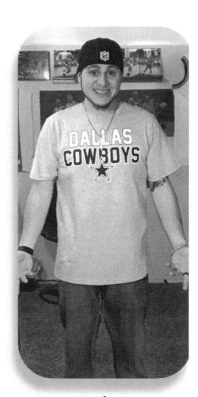

*Before*　　　　　　　　　　　　*After*

# TIME TO CRUSH IT!

**T**HANKS FOR STICKING with me through this book. I hope you're now feeling empowered to take your life back once and for all, by taking this new turn on your life's journey.

In parting, I want to leave you with a few tips to get the best possible, and most lasting, results for yourself.

**Reread this book once a month.** Immersing yourself in what works is key to both your initial and your ongoing success. It's like I said: You've spent decades immersed in the habits, choices and environments that got you where you are. It's going to take more than reading one book, one time, to get and keep you headed in this new direction. To think otherwise is the diet mentality at work and we already know that doesn't work, right?

**Stop, drop, and roll.** Make your list of 100 things that make you feel good. Then keep it someplace, like your phone, where you can easily find and reference it. Get in the habit of using your 100 things list to feel better, instead of resorting to food. It'll take some mindfulness, especially at first, but you can totally do it. It's SO worth it to feel that freedom from emotional eating.

**Get and stay connected to the Code Red Rebel community.** There are days when the pull of your old life is gonna be strong and when your willpower won't be enough. Those are the days when connection to a community can keep you from staying down if you fall down. (Plus you'll get a healthy hit of oxytocin when you hear about success stories or get support from your peers.)

I get it. Asking for and accepting help feels vulnerable. But asking for help doesn't make you weak and needing help doesn't mean there's anything wrong with you. All it means is that you're a human being. Heck, I ask for help all the time—from my family, my staff, my friends and coaches I work with. There aren't enough hours in the day for me to figure everything out myself. By not asking for help, I'd lose valuable time, waste a lot of energy and go without the outcome I want.

Plus, having those like-minded people around is HUGE. The world is full of environments and people that will tempt you to go back to wasn't working. Even rationalize it. Those are the times you lean on your like-minded community to stay immersed in what DOES work.

Remember: It doesn't matter who you are or what you do. You can follow this lifestyle and take your life back. This book is not for one type of person. It's for everyone, including YOU.

You can do this. You DESERVE IT.

Cristy Code Red

P.S. I love hard work. Yet as hard as I work, I can't make a revolution happen by myself. It takes people - lots of people - speaking up and being the example.

That's where you come in. Live the Code Red Lifestyle. Show 'em how it's done.

Share this book with someone who needs it. Review this book. Talk about it.

You can reach people I'll never be able to reach.

***Together, we can change the world!***

APPENDIX

# ADDITIONAL SUCCESS STORIES

Nancy Bond
Lewiston, Idaho
Age 57
Lost 65 pounds

I was fairly thin my whole life. I always had this chubby little face, but I was slim and athletic. I ate all the time though, even in high school. It was horrible stuff, like fast food.

I was 24 when I had my daughter. The pregnancy was very rough and sadly we lost her identical twin. Afterwards, I just ate whatever I felt like and put on 90 pounds. Then the depression set in. I was extremely miserable during that time and got up to 250 pounds.

Then I joined Nutrisystem. A year later, I'd lost about 65 pounds, but I never could lose the last 20 pounds that I wanted to. Of course, I gained it back and began that cycle of yo-yo dieting. I'd put on 40 to 50 pounds, try some program, lose some weight, and then put it right back on. I never could figure out why I kept doing that. I always felt bad about myself.

My health suffered. I'd had debilitating gout in my feet for 20 years.

Sometimes it was so bad I'd be unable to move for days, although I took medication for it. I've also had high cholesterol for 30-plus years, ever since my daughter was born. When I say high, I mean HIGH—in the 400s. No medication I tried could get it out of that range. It was so bad, I could have had a heart attack at any moment. It was just so high and my doctors couldn't control it.

I've also had Type II diabetes since I was 38. Right before Code Red, I was on the highest dose of medicine I could take for it without being on an insulin pump. I was even in the beginning stages of chronic kidney failure. At 40, I had my gallbladder removed.

I didn't realize I was a sugar addict, because if you put a piece of bread and a piece of cake in front of me, I'd go for the bread and eat the whole loaf. As a diabetic, that was dangerous. The scariest part is that I had no idea how much sugar I was really taking in, and here's why: The "diabetic diet" I was taught to eat didn't allow sugar in obvious forms like desserts, yet I was encouraged to eat bread and pasta.

I couldn't get up without my bones aching. Every joint hurt. It would take me a few minutes to get walking because my hips were just killing me, not to mention my feet and my knees. It was horrible. I remember looking at a picture of myself from a vacation I took to St. Thomas and thinking,

*How did I get this heavy again? What can I do about it? There's got to be something out there that works.*

In 2017, we hosted a barbecue. My friend Becky and her husband, Jeff, came over. She and I had both struggled with weight loss for years. We'd go to the gym two hours a day, yet still we couldn't conquer our weight. When I saw Becky at that barbecue, she looked happy. Becky had been on the Code Red Lifestyle for a couple of months and she looked good.

Looking into the program, part of me thought, *Yeah, it looks easy, but it's gotta be hard*. I didn't think I could succeed, because up until that point I'd consistently failed at diets. I kept watching Becky and when a Holiday Hustle Challenge came up, I thought, *Well, maybe it will work for me*. Maybe it would have, if I'd tried harder. Just getting the water down was hard. I was used to drinking 6 to 12 cans of Diet 7-Up a day. I'd been doing that for the last 10 years.

Even though I had bombed in the Holiday Hustle, I decided to give the next challenge a shot—a 10 Pound Takedown. I tried a lot harder. My daughter-in-law Leisha joined me, and that really helped. In my other weight-loss attempts, I didn't have the support system of the group. That challenge flipped a switch for me. I realized I needed more, so I invested in a custom program. After that, I didn't falter at all.

The first week—during detox—I was pretty miserable. I got angry at the drop of a hat. Because I went from drinking a 12-pack of Diet 7-Up a day to a gallon of water instead, my body bloated like nobody's business. I put on 10 pounds the first couple of days. My body had no idea what to do with all that water.

On the eighth day, everything changed. I felt like a totally different person. I had more energy. I had lost all the weight I'd put on while my body adjusted to the water and my weight just kept dropping. That's when I realized I could do it.

I'd never had that certainty and confidence before. Ever since I was a little kid, for some reason, I never felt quite good enough. I took that feeling into my adult life. I felt like I wasn't good enough to lose weight and feel good about myself. Joining Code Red helped me finally accept that I am worthy of losing weight and being happy.

I was surprised to learn how grains turned to sugar during digestion— how they were about the worst food to eat for someone with Type II diabetes. Adjusting to Code Red-approved food wasn't hard. I got to eat bacon and butter! I was used to avoiding both on other programs because I was told they were bad for me, that they caused high cholesterol and that I'd die if I kept eating them.

When I got down to my goal weight of 145, I thought, *Wow, this is sustainable for me! I haven't weighed 145 for 30 years. I feel accomplished, and that feels wonderful.*

Maintenance is sometimes a little challenging for me. I've had my slip-ups. One Frito can become a whole bag pretty quickly. Fortunately, with the Code Red Lifestyle™, it's easy to get right back on track.

Cristy's "What's Eating You?" online course helped me figure out why I was struggling in moments like those. Staying connected to Code Red and having that support system makes it easier to get back on track if you have a bad day.

In the past, that's where I always failed—after I lost my weight. Having the support system and knowing what to do when I faltered made all the difference.

My husband was a medical doctor for 30 years—his training told him you can't eat the kind of stuff I was eating and lose weight and be healthy. In his experience, the way I was eating would kill me. He was sure I was drinking too much water. Fortunately, he's not the kind of person who will tell me what to do. As I persisted with Code Red, he simply watched me. As the weight melted off and my lab results improved, he saw how much better I felt and he came around. Now he's pretty good about hiding his snacks from me and he eats Code Red-approved foods most of the time. He's been a great support.

One night, I came home from a long day at work. It was late, but I needed something to eat. He looked at me and said, "Ain't nobody gonna die from skipping a meal," pointing to our refrigerator magnet with that quote on it.

He's even said he wished he knew about Code Red when he was practicing medicine, remarking "I would have had all of my heavy patients on it."

Leisha, my daughter-in-law, is my Code Red buddy. We check in with each other every day—she was my biggest support during my journey. Being able to email my coach helped too. Between my coaching group and the Code Red LIFE group, I never felt like I was alone. When I felt down, I could rely on them to lift me up. Those communities and Leisha are why I'm still successful now and why I'll never go back.

When I started the Code Red Lifestyle, most of my coworkers thought I was super crazy. Many insisted it wasn't safe to drink so much water (even though they didn't have an issue with all the 7-Up I was drinking). Instead of letting them get to me, I let the naysayers motivate me, determined to show them this was safe—that not only would I succeed, but so could they.

They watched my progress. I'm not a pusher, but when people had questions, I'd suggest they read *The Code Red Revolution*. At least 20 people at work joined Code Red because they saw what I accomplished with it. One of my biggest naysayers saw my success, sold all her Isagenix products, joined Code Red, and lost 60 pounds.

People I know are losing weight left and right. I love it.

My health is so much better I can hardly believe it! My gout, high cholesterol, Type II diabetes, aches and pains are GONE. I have so much energy, I bounce out of bed in the morning like a little kid. Who would have thought that in my 50s, all these problems would go away just by eating real food?

Before Code Red, I would have never thought that was possible. It leads you to the root of your problems, identifying the part of you that wants food for comfort. The "diets" I tried in the past didn't address any of that. Code Red is the whole package. It's been such a privilege to be a part of this revolution.

If you're thinking about trying the Code Red Lifestyle, take the leap. Do it. Even if you're in your 50s like me, do it. Life's too short to spend it feeling miserable. Figure out why you want to do this and do it. It will work if you follow the rules.

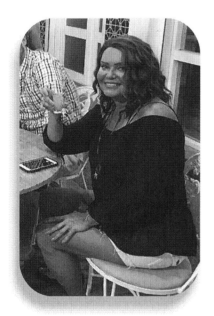 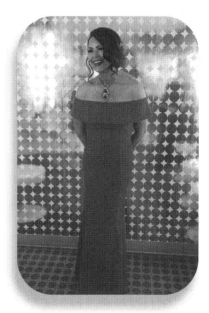

*Before*          *After*

Natasha Hazlett
Franklin, Tennessee
Age 41
Lost 55.5 pounds

I remember the day I contacted Cristy like it was yesterday. I had hit rock bottom. I could not stand to look at myself in the mirror anymore. That day started with me in tears, but I ended it with a huge smile, because I made a decision that I knew would change my life forever.

My disordered eating started at the age of 13. My family members are all thin people, so I put a lot of pressure on myself to be thin like them even though I had a bigger frame. I took diet pills and joined weight-loss programs like Jenny Craig and Nutrisystem—when I probably didn't even need to.

As a result of the diet roller coaster, I had an unhealthy relationship with food. I'd eat a ton for a few weeks, and then go on a diet. Then I'd eat a ton again, gain the weight back (and then some), and go on the next diet. By the time I got engaged, I was at my heaviest—I had gained 30 pounds since graduating from law school.

To prepare for my wedding, I started the Body For Life program, which had a nutrition component and a strict exercise regimen. It was awful because I don't like going to the gym. But since this was my wedding, I sucked it up and did the program. I hated every second of it, but I hit my goal weight.

After the wedding, I was totally done with diets. I had been on one diet or another since I was 13 and never wanted to think about my weight ever again. I decided that I was entitled to splurge because of my 14 years of dieting. Unfortunately, I "splurged" my way from a size 8 to a size 16/18.

My seven-year infertility struggle only exacerbated the situation, because I used food to deal with that disappointment. I eventually ballooned up to 210 pounds. I can't express how ashamed I felt. I used to love to go shopping, but it became a chore I dreaded because I was continually buying clothes in bigger sizes. It was humiliating. After each trip to the store, I hated myself even more.

At that point I said, "Ok, Natasha. You've got to do something. This is getting out of control." So I put myself through 17 weeks of the South Beach Diet. After feeling hungry and deprived the whole time, I only lost 23 of the 60 pounds I had gained. The thought of having to suffer through another 6 months was unbearable. So I quit and went back to my old habits.

My spiral toward the bottom started as I was planning my daughter's first birthday party. I was looking for pictures of me and my daughter to use at the party. I could barely find any! I couldn't believe how hard it was to find photos of the two of us together—this beautiful baby I had prayed for and waited so long for.

That's when I realized it was because I was ashamed of my size. I didn't want to be in the pictures, because I didn't want to "ruin" them by being so fat. I feared that one day she would come to me and say, "Mommy, why aren't there any pictures of us when I was little?" What was I supposed to tell her? That I was ashamed of who I was? Because that was the truth. That wasn't the example I wanted to set for my daughter.

The sad reality was that when I looked in the mirror, I hated the person staring back at me. It sounds terrible, but I hated her. All I could think was *Who is this person? This is not me! What happened to me?* I didn't want to go out with my friends because I didn't want to be the fat girl in the pictures. My business was suffering because I hated being on video, even though that's what I needed to do to continue growing it. I was in a really dark place.

Then I ran into a friend who I hadn't seen in about 5 months, and she had totally transformed herself. She had lost close to 60 pounds and looked completely different. She told me, "It's just an eating plan. No exercise." I couldn't believe what I was hearing!

I followed Cristy on Facebook for months before I finally reached out. "Okay, Cristy, let's do this. I'm ready to be the woman God intended me to be."

Because of my dramatic weight loss and the fact that I've kept it off, people want to do what I did. The funny thing is they keep saying, "Surely there are shakes to buy or pills to take, right? What about expensive food to buy?" I just say "NO! Just follow the simple rules and you'll get the results."

Once I signed up for a program with Cristy and I got the rules, I read them over and over thinking *That's it?! Really? How can this be possible?* The rules really are that simple. You just follow them and you lose weight.

No one had ever told me that I should skip the gym and get some extra sleep. It was so freeing to know I could eat real food and sleep and just live my life without taking pills, drinking shakes, or buying expensive, flavorless diet foods.

I lost 55 pounds in just over 5 months.

When people tell me, "You worked so hard for this. You deserve it," I almost feel guilty, because it wasn't hard. Sure, I missed chocolate a little, but I didn't have to go to the gym! The best part is that I now have the tools I need to stay healthy and trim forever. I can go on vacation and indulge. Then when I get home, I hop right back on the program and the 5 or 7 pounds I gained come right off! This is truly a lifestyle, not a diet.

The Code Red Lifestyle has truly made me a better mother, wife, business coach, and friend. Now I'm not afraid to hop into pictures or take videos for my business. The ripple effect has been amazing. Some of my closest friends have worked with Cristy, and their lives have been transformed as well. In fact, over 50 of my friends joined up on Cristy's latest challenge, and they're getting awesome results!

People ask me all the time, "Do you think this could work for me?" I just want to shout, "Yes! Yes! Yes! If you're vegan, this will work for you. If you're pregnant, this will work for you. If you're a man or a woman, old or young, if you travel all the time, or you like to eat out...it will work for you!

I am 100% certain that I'm never going back to where I was. Fat, unhealthy Natasha is just not who I am anymore. Although I struggled privately with my weight for years, I decided to share my story because I want to give a voice to people who are where I was—silently struggling with their weight. If you look in the mirror right now and hate yourself, I know how you feel. You are not alone. You can do this, I promise. It's easy. It just works.

YOU CAN TAKE YOUR LIFE BACK.

I should know...because I did.

## 4 YEAR UPDATE

Since 2017, I was able to get pregnant and give birth to twins, then lose over 50 pounds after they were born. My twins were full-term and healthy, and my pregnancy was perfect. And I know this was because of the Code Red

Lifestyle, where I learned to care for my body, eat nourishing food, drink enough water and get plenty of sleep.

I sought to uncover the reason I struggled with my weight in the first place. As a result, I was able to let go of self-hatred, lack of self-worth, lack of confidence—everything that had held me back from who I was divinely designed to be. I call it the "unbecoming process," from this saying I love: "Maybe the journey isn't so much about becoming anything. Maybe it's about unbecoming everything that isn't really you, so you can be who you were meant to be in the first place."

A book was placed on my heart and as a result of going through the *unbecoming process,* I felt prepared to write it and did so in just 22 days! It's called *Unstoppable Influence: Be You. Be Fearless. Transform Lives.* As a result of writing that book and sharing it with the world, I've helped tens of thousands of people transform their lives. It all started with that decision to love myself again.

Once I became pregnant with twins, I hired someone who specializes in maternal nutrition for multiple pregnancies. It required me to eat food I hadn't eaten in two and a half years, which was emotionally difficult. But once the twins were a few months old, I got right back into the Code Red Lifestyle.

After I gave birth, many people outside the Code Red community tried to convince me it was okay not to lose the baby weight, but I didn't want to carry that weight around for years like I'd seen many others do.

We have an obesity epidemic in today's world and most people are content to be unhealthy, on medications and out of shape. Staying connected to a support system of like-minded individuals has definitely made a world of difference.

Code Red isn't complicated, nor is it a radical diet. It's a lifestyle. It's a different way of eating that is completely doable, whether you're sitting at home, traveling, or anything in between. I'm a married mother of three who runs her own business. Yet no matter what's happening in my life, the Code Red Lifestyle fits right into it.

Losing weight has been a constant battle for me. I gained a lot of weight after having kids and really just not paying attention to my body. I spent money on everything I could think of to lose weight. I worked out regularly, so I couldn't understand why it was so hard to stay healthy. Eventually, I got to the point where I just accepted that I was heavy and that was how it was going to be forever. I was definitely depressed. I didn't feel like myself.

I found Cristy's Code Red program online and wondered, *Why would this work? What makes this any different from the dozens of other diets we've tried?* Then I went upstairs and got ready for bed. The moment that stopped me in my tracks was when I had to squeeze into my pajama bottoms. I thought, *This is just ridiculous. I shouldn't have to work hard to pull my large PJs over my rear.*

That's when I'd just had enough. It was time to change.

I had tried and given up on so many different weight-loss methods and nothing had worked for very long. I knew several people who had been successful with Cristy. So I decided to trust what I saw with my own eyes and give it a try.

Being at rock bottom feels awful. I was desperate and didn't know what to expect. But meeting Cristy was so exciting. She explained everything so clearly and for the first time, I really had hope. I decided that it was time to take care of me. I was going to make this work no matter what. I actually took out a loan to get a personal program with Cristy and it was the best decision I ever made.

I used to eat until my stomach felt like it would burst. I was always taught to clean my plate no matter what. It was hard, but I learned to listen to my body and only eat when I was truly hungry. I get to eat real food that I can just go buy at the grocery store. No pills or shakes to order or buy.

I actually sleep now! I've got energy and I'm happy. I want to go places and do things. The transformation has been amazing. I feel like a different person.

The biggest surprise was that I wasn't hungry. Every diet I had tried worked okay...for a little while. Then came a holiday or a birthday party with cakes and cookies and other yummy food. It's much easier to ignore that stuff if you're not hungry.

You're not starving yourself on this program. It's easy to give up the stuff that makes you feel terrible. People ask me what pills I'm taking to lose weight and I tell them I'm not taking any. I mean, what are you going to do—take pills for the rest of your life? No! I'm on bacon and eggs. That's sustainable.

I started around 185 and now I'm down to 125. I thought I'd be lucky to get to 140. When I finally got to goal weight, it was such a shock!

The support from the Code Red community makes such a huge difference. Cristy fiercely believes that you can do this and she won't accept anything less than your best. These people are part of my family now.

I've been able to keep living a normal life while continuing to lose weight. I've even managed to keep losing while on vacation. That never happened on other programs. I took my food scale, measuring spoons and bathroom scale with me and just did what I had to do. Best of all, I still had fun!

The key is to be prepared. I cook my food ahead of time and bring it with me. I am never without my water bottle and little snacks like cashew butter and pepperoni sticks. Wherever I go, I am always prepared and never hungry.

It's weird how people get used to their pain. We get used to our joints hurting. We accept that we can't get to the top of the stairs without panting. We just push it to the back of our minds and go on with life, but those signs are our bodies warning us that we are unhealthy. Pay attention to those warning signs and do something.

Within a week or two of starting the Code Red Lifestyle, I really noticed the changes—particularly, how much better I was sleeping. When you take all the crap out of your diet, you wake up in the morning feeling refreshed. You feel like you actually got some sleep. None of the other programs I tried even mentioned sleep.

How can you put a price tag on your happiness and your health? I was prediabetic, but I'm not anymore. I had gastric problems—those are gone. I'm happy, healthy, and I have the tools to stay that way forever.

With this book, you have the tools in your hand. Trust the program. Follow the rules. Even if they don't make sense to you, or they're the opposite of what you've been told. Just trust Cristy. Read the success stories. If you're struggling with your weight, take a chance and try something different.

Take your life back. It doesn't get better than this!

**3-YEAR UPDATE**

Not much has changed for me since I lost my weight in 2016.

My lifestyle is the same. I've added exercise, but the way I eat hasn't changed.

A big part of my success in keeping my weight off is continuing to be connected to the Code Red community. I also still keep my meals simple, usually just three ingredients. I've continued to drink all my water and weigh every morning, just as Cristy instructs for weight maintenance.

My advice for lasting success on the Code Red Lifestyle is to stay connected. Continue to weigh every day, drink your water and keep junk food out of your house.

I know that if I don't stay in line, I will end up back where I was before Code Red. I do not ever want to be there again.

Ree Rote
Meridian, Idaho
Age 60
Lost 80 pounds in 7 months

In high school, I dieted, even though I wasn't actually fat. I was very curvy—big-busted, small waist, wide hips. I felt heavy, even though I wasn't, because I was also short. Through my 20s, I gained a little weight here and there, but my weight didn't become a problem until my 30s.

Back then, there weren't all these weight-loss shakes and very few diet pills. It was more about starvation. Don't eat breakfast, try not to eat anything all day, eat as little as possible. Of course that didn't work.

In college, I actually did try diet pills. They worked and worked quickly, but only until I stopped taking them. I also did Fen Phen when that was popular.

When the shakes started popping up, I tried several of those and they worked for a while. Everything works temporarily. I could do them for a short time, but finally I just couldn't take it anymore. Then I was stuck. What do I do now that I'm not drinking shakes for breakfast, lunch, and dinner?

I never learned anything about using good nutrition to lose weight. I only ever knew about quick fixes. They might get a little weight off, but they don't address why you're heavy in the first place.

Every time I tried to lose weight, I'd gain it right back. It felt like I was torturing myself. One minute I'd tell myself, "At least I can eat whatever I want. I'm healthy. My husband and family love me. I've got a good life. I like myself."

I didn't like that I was fat and couldn't wear cute clothes, but I liked myself. I thought maybe I should just give up and be a fat grandmother.

And then a little voice would say, "No, no. Don't give up. Try one more time."

Through the holidays that year, I was able to lose 15 pounds in three months on my own. I'd successfully dieted through the holidays before.

Right afterward, I immediately put on six pounds for the usual reason: I didn't want to deprive myself.

I actually knew Cristy before getting involved in the Code Red Lifestyle. I started hearing more and more about her, through friends who were enjoying success with her program. I began following her on Facebook. Seeing so many before-and-after photos of people who had lost more than 100 pounds was motivating. The bigger the person was, the more impressed I was, because I realized that if somebody that heavy could do it—somebody with more weight to lose than I did—then I could be successful, too.

I finally realized I couldn't do it by myself, so I joined the next 10 Pound Takedown Cristy offered. It was February 2018. By that time, I'd learned more about good nutrition. My husband and I had cleaned up our diet quite a bit, but I was still eating organic grains and pasta and other things we thought were healthy. I still didn't understand how to use nutrition to lose weight.

Early in the challenge, I really leaned on Cristy's certainty in her program. **Just a couple weeks in, I knew deep in my soul that I wasn't just going to lose "some" weight this time. I was going to lose it ALL.** I no longer had to lean on Cristy's certainty, because I finally had my own.

Then I was all in. Losing weight became a priority, almost like a job. There was no indecision or doubt. It was black and white for me: Follow the program, weigh myself, drink water. Simple!

I never cheated. When faced with the choice to eat a piece of candy or not, I didn't struggle with the decision. I'd already made the more powerful decision to stay on track no matter what.

Thankfully, I did not have to endure any naysayers. My husband even joined the challenge so he could support me. That made it even more fun. We'd get up each day and ask each other "What was your weight this morning?"

It was like a mini competition. Nothing serious, just enough motivation to make it fun. He's been a terrific support. In fact, my whole family has been deeply supportive.

I remember how amazing it felt to get into the 150s, even though I still had about 30 pounds until my goal weight. When I dieted on my own, the 160s were as low as I could get. As I got older, it got harder and harder to do.

So when I got into the 150s, it was familiar yet forgotten territory. I started to really feel good about how I looked. Goal weight felt even more incredible. People said I looked completely different. When I see old photos, I can't believe what I used to look like.

Now I wake up between 5:00 and 6:00 each morning with excitement and enthusiasm for the day—something I never did before Code Red. I can't wait to get out of bed and start the day.

Since reaching my goal, I realize the happiness I feel now goes beyond the emotional side of things. It's physical, because my body has so much more energy and my mind is clearer.

I really enjoy being able to cross my legs and sit comfortably. It feels very feminine and classy. I also love being able to wear beautiful clothes, because I was never able to do that before. I love being able to go into a nice store and have so many choices— not just settling for certain outfits because they're the only ones that fit.

Traveling is also so much easier now. I can carry my bags through the airport and down the aisle of a plane without worrying that I'm going to bump everyone with parts of my body. I can even sit in the middle seat now, because I have room on both sides of me. Before, I'd always want the aisle seat.

My only real struggle has been navigating maintenance. Don't get me wrong, maintenance is great. It has so much more flexibility than weight-loss mode. But because of that flexibility, my huge appetite comes into play. I can just eat and eat and eat, without so much as a stomachache.

What I've learned is that, though I rarely feel full, I do feel satiated. **By listening to my body, exactly the way Cristy teaches us, I've been able to figure out when to stop eating.** Weighing myself every morning helps me stay ahead of my appetite as well.

Inspiring other people is immensely rewarding. When someone comes up to me and says, "I'm doing this because of you," it gives me goosebumps. It's one of my favorite parts of being a Code Red Rebel.

So many of my family members have joined Code Red challenges because of pictures I posted. They'd seen me lose weight before only to gain it back. But when I got to a certain point, they were like, "Wow, okay, if she can do this, I can do it!" It's amazing that these people are all changing their lives just because they've seen me do it.

I have a cousin who got lap-band surgery and still couldn't lose the weight, but she joined the 10 Pound Takedown and is thinner now than she's been her entire life. So many of these people are also getting off medications.

All that motivates me more now than ever to keep myself healthy so other people will continue to be inspired and change their lives. I want everybody else to experience what I've experienced with the Code Red Lifestyle.

When I look back now, I could smack my high school self for thinking I was fat. In fact, today at goal weight, I weigh exactly what I weighed in high school! I am healthier now than I was then.. I have more energy and enthusiasm and I feel so much better!

Staying connected to the Code Red LIFE group is so valuable. It keeps you accountable and encouraged. I found that to encourage others, I need to be doing well too. Plus keeping myself visible in the group helped me feel accountable and stay motivated.

Anyone who's thinking about joining the Code Red Lifestyle knows they have a problem and that they can't fix it on their own. Join a 10 Pound Takedown and see how encouraging and simple it is. It's not always easy, but the program is so simple.

Sometimes you see dramatic results and you think, "Oh gosh, I'm going to have to change everything." There will be some changes, but you're still eating real food. The simplicity of implementing Code Red, the encouragement of the group and the continued education gives you the skills and knowledge you need to be successful.

**If you could just feel for a moment how it feels to be at your goal weight, you'd realize that every struggle along the way will be worth it.** In the meantime, lean on the certainty of people who've already succeeded.

One day, like me, you'll start to believe it too!

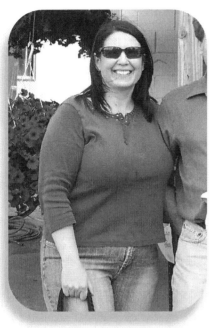

*Before*

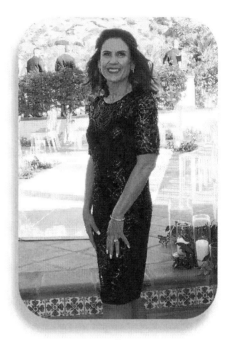

*After*

Sheli Fulcher-Koontz
Star, Idaho
Age 52
Lost 35 pounds

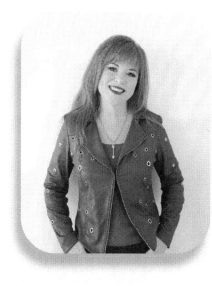

My weight-loss story is different from most. I'm only about 5' 2", and growing up I was always petite. Even into early adulthood, I never had any trouble keeping in shape. I certainly never thought I needed to lose weight, let alone that someday I would tell a weight-loss story.

My struggle with weight began when I became a mother. I had my child later than most people do and I never got all the baby weight off. On top of that, I love to eat. I thought maybe the little switch in my brain that's supposed to tell me I'm full was broken.

My family has a history of pretty severe high cholesterol. I was working with an endocrinologist on gene therapy to manage it and he told me that the likelihood of my having a cardiac event wasn't a matter of *if*, but *when*. When a doctor says that you will have a heart attack or a stroke at some point, it really grabs your attention!

I can eat a lot. When I got into my 40s, I was eating like someone in their teens or 20s and it caught up with me. I never felt fat unless I saw a picture of myself or looked in a mirror. When I did that, I hated what I saw.

My first attempts to lose weight were not successful, partly because I wasn't committed to whatever I was doing at the time. I would lose 5 or 10 pounds, but then I would stop and gain it back. I always justified it though. I told myself that I was just at "that age" where people gain weight.

I met Cristy through a group of professionals in my community called the Rockstar Network and was immediately intrigued. She has this incredible presence. I took one look at her and wondered, *What's her story?* She was very kind and engaging, so I followed her on Facebook.

Months later, I decided I had to try something for the sake of my health. Even though I hadn't been successful with weight loss before, I took the leap and signed up for a one-on-one program. It was a lot of money, but that investment made me take the program seriously.

The program was simple, but at the same time difficult. One of our sayings in the Code Red family is "Pick your hard." The program was hard, but walking around waiting for a heart attack was harder. I needed to do it and I am so grateful that I did.

I started my program on December 1. I was not prepared for the lack of support from people who I thought would be in my corner. Someone actually asked me, "How could you be so dumb to start a weight-loss program during the holidays?" I was shocked. Another person asked, "What are you going to do when you gain it all back?"

Looking back, I realize they were heavy themselves and not ready to make the change in their lives so they felt the need to tear me down, but Code Red shows you that you are stronger than you think.

The support from Cristy and the Code Red family has been simply outstanding. When you're making a lifestyle change like this one, it's worth more than gold to have a support group you can take your fears or struggles to. Cristy is really good at helping you "field the haters," so to speak.

Thanks to this group, when that person accused me of being dumb for starting a weight-loss program during the holidays, I was able to smile and say, "If I can be successful through the holidays, then I know I can be successful the rest of the time too."

I've built amazing relationships among the Code Red Rebels. I've made friends with so many wonderful people who I wouldn't have met otherwise, all looking out for each other. One woman needed to go shopping for "regular-sized" clothes, which she had never done before. I met her at the mall and supported her on this part of her journey. We had so much fun! That kind of support helps this program stand out from others.

I won't lie—the first week was horrible. I never thought I had a sugar addiction, but detoxing off sugar is a terrible experience. Quitting Diet Coke, bread, and pasta was not easy. I whined and complained, but Cristy was tough with me. Patient, but firm. I needed her to be like that, because I have a strong personality myself. She and I were a good match.

Cristy is so encouraging. During the first week, she kept telling me, "Wait until Day 8—you'll feel like you've woken up." She was right. Day 8 finally rolled around and I felt incredible. The headaches were gone, I had no pain and I wasn't craving junk food at all. From that day forward, I did everything Cristy said. She monitored me, kept me on track and battled with me when needed to make sure I was successful.

Then I started to notice that others seemed to lose more weight faster than me. I'm naturally competitive, so I wanted to lose two to five pounds a week like the other Rebels. I also didn't have as much to lose. My 35-pound journey was someone else's 60 or 100-pound journey. Cristy helped me see that comparing myself to someone else was devastating to my morale. I had to learn that any loss I had was progress and that there was nothing wrong with me—my journey was just different.

My family was great. My dad has been my #1 cheerleader, to an embarrassing point. He tells others about my weight loss because he's so proud. My husband was worried about my health, so he's happy for the improvement in my life. He chooses not to eat the way I do, but that's fine. My ten-year-old son was my little accountability manager. He met Cristy and was very taken with her. From then on, he was always there to make sure I stayed on track. Whenever he thought I was going to cheat or have something I shouldn't, he'd say, "Don't you eat that. It's not Code Red Approved. I have Cristy's number!" He was great.

Now, my son doesn't need to lose any weight, but he does have ADHD. So I adjusted what he eats a little bit. Nothing extreme, just fewer carbs and less sugar with more fat and protein. Just that little tweak has really improved his behavior and attention.

At this point, I am 35 pounds down. I haven't been this small since I was 18! In addition to once again wearing a one-digit dress size, I got good news from my doctor. My cholesterol dropped 100 points! And that's while I was eating eggs, bacon, avocado, and coconut oil. After that, I went back to my endocrinologist and told him the news. I expected him to be concerned about what I was eating, but he just said, "Whatever you're doing, it's working. Keep it up." I no longer have to take Glucophage for prediabetes.

I do things now that I couldn't before. I was a den mother for the Cub

Scouts and am now involved with Scouts BSA with my son. I can hike 15 miles with the kids when I used to only manage three or four. I can walk up a hill or a flight of stairs without seeing stars. I can look in a mirror without feeling revulsion.

I didn't realize how much I hated myself until I made this lifestyle change. They say we're our own worst critics and that was so true for me. I used to call myself horrible names that I would never call anyone else. Now I have a new appreciation for myself.

Cristy talks about "taking your life back." With her help, that is exactly what I did. It wasn't easy, but it wasn't any harder than hating what I saw in the mirror every day. I did it because I *could* do it. You can too.

### 3-Year Update

Wow, what *hasn't* changed in the past three years? In addition to remaining tight with the Code Red community, I merged my solo law practice into a larger firm, learned an additional area of law and became a partner. I am now the mother of a teenage boy—yikes!

All of this change would have been much more challenging had I not conquered my weight loss and my toxic relationship with food. Reaching my goal weight and keeping it off since March 2017 has allowed many doors to open in my life that would have been far too scary to walk through had I not already proven to myself that I can do hard things.

Now I use the confidence and knowledge I gained from Code Red to serve others, especially other Rebels. It doesn't get much better than that!

I naively thought that going into maintenance meant life would be problem-free from a food standpoint. Nope! That's when the "mental" work began. I had to understand and treat my toxic relationship with food so that I didn't revert to my old ways and gain the weight back.

I had to learn what weight-loss sustainability means and how to achieve it without yo-yo-ing in and out of it. I still have the same temptations, stress, and uncertainties that everyone else does. Choosing to stay Code Red-compliant gives me freedom and I feel so much better when I'm eating healthy.

When I reached maintenance, I approached it from a scientific standpoint. I became my own lab rat. Through a lot of experimentation, I determined which foods I could reintroduce, how often I could eat them and which choices I should avoid.

I tested every Code Red rule too and found several that made maintenance easy. I now schedule, on a monthly basis, what and when to have something non-Code Red-compliant.

It's pretty simple.

Get on the scale every day so you can quickly course-correct if something is off.

Drink the recommended amount of water every day.

Do not allow junk food to infiltrate your house. It's not the 50 times you make it past the temptation successfully; it's the fifty-first time that will get you!

Realize that food will not fix crisis or stress. Get real about your emotional eating. Code Red offers so many great resources to heal your toxic relationship with food.

This structure and plan are key to keeping my weight off. There's no flying by the seat of my (now much smaller) pants!

Yvette Price
Orofino, Idaho
Age 75
Lost 75 pounds in 7 months, right before she turned 75

At the age of seven, I had my tonsils removed. I started putting on weight afterward and it became a lifelong battle. It wasn't until I hit my mid-60s that I ended up in a wheelchair.

At the time, my doctor told me I would never walk again, but he didn't explain why I needed to be in a wheelchair. I figured that if physical therapy or something else would have helped me, surely my doctor would have said so.

My health deteriorated. I had Type 2 diabetes and was on insulin. I also had high cholesterol and high blood pressure. Of course I was on a special diet for my diabetes, but it wasn't helping much and it included a lot of snacking.

Over the years, I had tried many different diets, including high-protein and Atkins, to get my weight off, but none of them worked like I hoped. My weight got as high as 275 pounds.

I found the Code Red Lifestyle through my daughter, Denice. At that time, I weighed 206, which was a lot on my petite frame. Denice had won a 10 Pound Takedown Challenge in June of 2017, then started a custom program and lost 68 pounds. It was encouraging to see her lose so much weight so quickly.

She would bring me food to try that she was eating and gave me a copy of Cristy's *Code Red Cookbook*. That got me hooked on Code Red. The food was so good!

I was taught that I couldn't have real butter and that full-fat sour cream or cottage cheese were unhealthy. To be able to eat those things while losing weight and healing from disease was thrilling! Plus I was so much more satisfied eating all those healthy fats. It felt like a treat.

I was pleasantly surprised to learn I didn't need as much protein as I'd thought. Cristy wants you to eat your vegetables and I love that because

I've always been a veggie eater. Being diabetic at that time, I was already staying away from sweets, so that part wasn't hard for me. To this day, I still don't miss them.

I can't tell you what a huge relief it was knowing I did not have to exercise. In fact, if having to exercise had been a requirement of losing my weight with Code Red, I would not have been successful. Because of my condition, I wouldn't have been able to anyway.

Once I made my mind up, I was vigilant about following the rules. It's simply food over hand—don't put it in your hand and it won't go in your mouth!

The way Code Red has affected my health has been nothing short of miraculous. Within four or five months of starting the lifestyle, I was able to stop taking seven of the nine medications I was on, including those for high blood pressure and Type II diabetes. Cristy teaches us not to snack between meals and when I stopped snacking it helped my diabetes so much. My doctor even put a note in my file: "Keep up the Code Red!" My vision has even improved...at the age of 75! I never dreamed that was possible. I had been going to the doctor every three months, but now I only have to go once a year.

When Denice brought me some of her shirts to wear, I told her, "Oh, they're not going to fit me." I was shocked when they did.

Denice took me to the doctor after I'd been on Code Red a few months, I asked them to please weigh me as soon as we got there. The nurse said, "No one ever *asks* to be weighed!" I was at 131, which I hadn't weighed since I was 12. I cried tears of joy.

Since losing my weight and healing my body with Code Red, I can stand for at least five minutes and I'm working on more each day. Because I'm so much lighter and I'm getting stronger, I can get all the way to my feet using only one hand. I can even transfer myself from my wheelchair to another chair. I've switched from a power wheelchair to a regular one that I move by turning the wheels. I put my feet on the floor and scoot myself around.

Best of all, I've made up my mind that I'm going to walk again!

I have no fear about maintaining my weight loss. Sometimes I'll have an apple or an orange, but most of the time I stick with Code Red-approved foods. I'm still drinking my water. I'm still waiting five hours between meals and I'm still eating two meals a day, because I'm completely satisfied with that.

Staying connected to Cristy and the Code Red community is a huge inspiration for me and for Denice. Sometimes I laugh, sometimes I cry... and sometimes Cristy is a little scary, but she's always inspiring. Plus hearing Cristy and other Code Red Rebels say, "We're here for you, you can do this, you're gonna do this!" helps a lot. Cristy encourages you so much and helps you believe you can do it. She encourages you to believe in yourself and that makes a big difference.

Having Denice on the journey with me helps so much too. She's my inspiration! She has inspired others too. Her husband and daughter have both lost weight with Code Red. Her daughter is now pregnant with my first great-grandchild, and I'm looking forward to babysitting.

I love talking to other people about Code Red. I get questions all the time. My UPS delivery man asked me about it. Denice and I told him about *The Code Red Revolution* book. He bought a copy and started watching Cristy online and now he's down 60 pounds!

On my seventy-fifth birthday, Cristy called me and filmed it live. It has inspired many people to join the program. I tell people that Code Red is the way to go because it's something that's good for you and you learn to control yourself. Mind over matter. I love Code Red and I love how I feel.

When you're overweight you feel helpless. When you are in a wheelchair as well, it can leave you feeling lost and powerless. Thanks to Code Red, I feel like I *do* have control and I *do* have a purpose, especially with my first great-grandbaby on the way. I'm looking forward to helping them learn to walk, holding them and even babysitting. Before Code Red, I wouldn't have been able to do all those things.

I want Cristy to keep doing what she's doing because she's changing lives. My family and I appreciate her.

If you're wondering whether to try Code Red, I want you to go for it! There's nothing out there like it. You'll end up so satisfied with your life, because it not only changes your body, it changes your attitude, your mindset—everything. It's awesome.

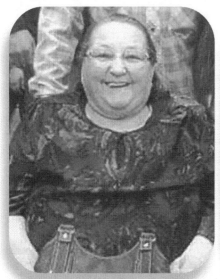 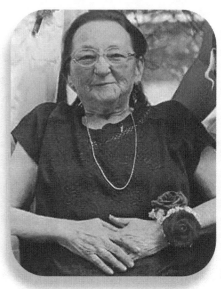

*Before* *After*

CRISTY "CODE RED" NICKEL has been in the health and fitness industry since 1994. In 2002, she began fighting as a professional boxer to earn money for college and became one of the most dangerous females on the planet. Cristy was featured on MTV's MADE, magazine covers, and other media outlets, even earning the title of "New York's Best Trainer" from Allure Magazine. After struggling with her own weight as a "fat athlete," Cristy created the Code Red Lifestyle to help overweight people get healthy with real food, water and sleep. Upon the release of her best selling book, "The Code Red REVOLUTION," Code Red exploded into an 8-figure company in only 3½ years, landing Cristy on huge stages and becoming one of the fastest growing entrepreneurs in the country. In 2024, Generation Iron released a worldwide documentary called "Cristy Code Red" about her life. Cristy splits her time between the city and mountains. She has a passion for weightlifting, snowboarding and running with her dog, Hazel.

## FOLLOW CRISTY

YouTube: www.CodeRed.tv

Instagram: @cristycodered

Facebook: www.facebook.com/CodeRedLifestyle

Twitter: @cristycodered

Code Red App: www.CodeRedLifestyle.com/App

Rebel Weight Loss & Lifestyle Podcast:
www.CodeRedLifestyle.com/Podcast

Made in United States
Troutdale, OR
09/23/2024